Aromatherapy for Everyone

*Discover the Scents of Health and
Happiness with Essential Oils*

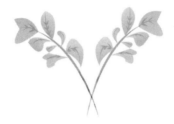

PJ Pierson
Mary Shipley

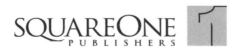

SQUAREONE
PUBLISHERS

BOOK DESIGN: Barbara Nice-Miller

Square One Publishers
115 Herricks Road
Garden City Park, NY 11040
(516) 535-2010 • (877) 900-BOOK
www.squareonepublishers.com

Printed in the United States of America

14

CONTENTS

This book is dedicated to Todd, Purrscilla, and Lucy, who love me no matter how I smell. Their very existance in my world makes life aromatically wonderful.

--Pamela Pierson

To Ann and J.T. for their love and support, John Moore and Nick Rana for their encouragement and Lou DeMers for his expertise.

--Mary Shipley

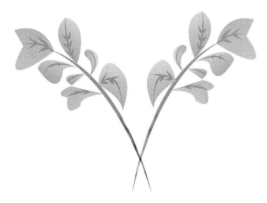

FOREWORD

The use of essential oils has literally been around for centuries. Not only do people derive a myriad of health benefits from these essential oils, but also a great deal of pleasure. The use of essential oils - or as it is known today, aromatherapy - is appealing because of their user-friendly nature, versatility and most significantly, their sensual properties.

Aromatherapy is a non-invasive way to take control of your health. Used in addition to other practices such as traditional Western medicine, yoga, meditation, diet, exercise or holistic medicine, aromatherapy can strengthen your overall health, well-being and vitality. Because of its growing acceptance with Americans, essential oils are now available almost anywhere you look. This is both good and bad news: good, because it's now easier for you to incorporate aromatherapy into your life and bad because, for the most part, these essential oils don't come with instructions.

In this book, we will help demystify aromatherapy by explaining its history and usage. We will also cover the basic essential oils, including their properties and therapeutic values. We'll also point out how to pick out a quality essential oil, and help you pick out a starter kit. You'll also learn about combining oils for synergistic blends, and the different ways aromatherapy can be incorporated into your life.

We firmly believe in the power of aromatherapy to strengthen us both physically and mentally. We've experienced this power for ourselves, and want to introduce it to you in an easy-to-understand way. After reading this book, we're positive you'll find yourself excited about the positive changes you can make in your life through aromatherapy.

With a little bit of guidance, you'll be able to safely and confidently integrate essential oils into your every day life. As we like to say, it will be a *scentsational* new lifestyle you'll embrace and enjoy. We can't wait for you to get started!

- Pamela Pierson and Mary Shipley

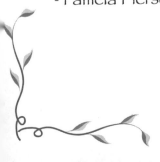
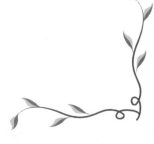

THE POWER
OF AROMATHERAPY

Aromatherapy. You may not know exactly what it is, but you can't escape it. Everywhere you turn, there is a plethora of scented candles, oils, sprays and incense all claiming to be good for your health and well-being. "Smell this and feel calm!" "Light this, and light his fire!" "Rub this scented lotion on your skin and re-energize your spirit!" Sounds like a bunch of nonsense just to sell products, doesn't it?

Strangely enough, it's not nonsense. In fact, there is more to aromatherapy than meets the nose. The use of scent to alter health and well-being for the better has been around for centuries. Now, science has confirmed what men and women have practiced for generations: scents have the ability to promote good physical, mental, and spiritual health. But how do you include aromatherapy in your everyday life? Is it easy? Does it make sense? And what exactly is it, anyway? This book will answer those questions, and more. Armed with the answers, you can change your life - and your health - for the better!

The Power of Aromatherapy

Have you ever been in a funk and then smelled something wonderful, like lavender or citrus, and suddenly felt better? That's the basis of aromatherapy. Essentially aromatherapy is a gentle, non-invasive, natural healing art that utilizes the scents of essential oils to promote general well-being. While essential oils do, in fact, have medicinal properties, the simple act of smelling an essential oil can uplift the spirit, which can positively change feelings and outlook.

The power of aromatherapy lies in its ability to stimulate the imagination and to generate an almost instant sense of joy or peace. And, unlike other therapies, such as acupuncture or traditional Western methods, aromatherapy is non-invasive. That means, nothing to take internally, no needles, no pain. It's also portable, so if you have recurring problems with stress, anxiety, migraines and the like, just take the applicable essential oil with you, and you have help right at the tip of your nose at all times.

Don't let all that New Age talk fool you: aromatherapy is not just a touchy-feely, warm fuzzy type of practice; there is most definitely science behind it. Aromatherapy falls under a fairly new science called *psychoneuroimmunology*, which studies the interaction among the psychological, neurological and immunological systems. In layman's terms, psychoneuroimmunology looks at the effects of both positive and negative experiences on the immune system and the psyche. Science has confirmed that pleasurable experiences like breathing in pleasant aromas or receiving a pampering massage actually strengthens the body's immune system and uplifts the spirit. Conversely, things like unhappiness, lack of touch and stale air lowers the body's resistance to disease and also dulls the spirit. So, incorporating aromatherapy into your daily activities can actually help bolster your immune system and promote a positive, clear outlook on life.

You may have heard of holistic medicine, which looks at the causes and prevention of illness, and not just the symptoms. It's a whole-body approach to health, one which gives you responsibility and a certain amount of control over your health. Aromatherapy is part of holistic medicine. When married to a healthy diet and lifestyle, it's a fabulous, sensual and creative way to keep on top of your health.

When did Aromatherapy arrive on the scene?

The way aromatherapy is all the talk these days, you'd think it was a brand new concept in health and wellness. It's not. It's almost as old as time itself.

While there is reason to believe that the use of aromatics has been in place since the dawn of mankind, physical evidence dates back to the ancient Egyptians. Clay tablets have been found that record the importation of cedarwood and cypress into Egypt and confirms the role essential oils played in international trade. Egyptian high priests also recorded the many uses of essential oils on to papyrus. One intriguing fact is that Imhotep, King Zoser's chief architect, renowned physician and astronomer, is also known as "the grandfather of aromatherapy." This great physician is credited with significant advances in medical knowledge. He regularly incorporated the use of aromatics into his practice.

Other cultures have used aromatics as well. The Chinese used aromatic herbs and massage well before the birth of Christ. The Indian therapy known as Ayurvedic medicine utilizes massage techniques, pressure points and essential oils to bring about good health. Hippocrates, the

Greek physician known as "The Father of Medicine," also promoted the daily use of aromatic baths and massage. These are just a few historical examples; the list also includes ancient Romans, various religious orders in the Middle Ages and continues through the centuries to these modern times.

Why do aromatics work?

It's not enough to know that aromatherapy has been around for ages, we also want to know *why* aromatics work. It doesn't seem possible that something as simple as the soothing smell of an essential oil could work wonders on health and well-being, yet it is not only possible, it happens because it utilizes our strongest sense: our sense of smell.

Of all five senses, sense of smell hits the brain first. Faster than a speeding bullet, it's the "Superman of Senses" with a direct path to the brain. Unlike many of our other senses, the olfactory system's nerve fibers do not pass through the "switching station," known as the dorsal thalmus. Instead, these nerve fibers run directly to the limbic area of the brain, which connects to the thalmus and neo-cortex. While these words may not have any meaning to you, this bit of information is important because it's how aromas are able to affect conscious thought and reactions. The limbic system links directly to our memories, stored learned responses, emotions and feelings.

Even though the olfactory system is linked directly to the brain, olfactory also involves other body systems as well. For example, someone breathing in an essential oil like peppermint not only absorbs it through the nasal cavity, but may also absorb it through the bronchial tract or lungs. This causes the essential oil molecules to pass into the body's circulatory system, increasing its benefits.

There is also an additional, and sensual, way to engage in aromatherapy: through the skin. This is done usually through massage, which has three very distinct benefits: that of touch, smell, and absorption. Essential oils can also be used in the bathtub, another relaxing and pampering activity. Besides being able to smell the essential oils being used on the skin, the extremely small molecules pass through the epidermis to the dermis, the layer of the skin that gives it its pliability. From there, the oil molecules pass into capillaries and into the rest of the circulatory system.

The body is not harmed by absorbing essential oils. The oils are expelled from the body in a variety of natural ways, like sweat, exhalation and so on. The length of time it takes to expel these oils varies from 3-14 hours, depending on the health of the body.

Essential oils do come with some warnings. One is do not use them directly on the eyes or the delicate mucous membranes of the body.

How do I use essential oils?

Aromatherapy is user-friendly, so there is no excuse to shy away from it. Once you understand a few basics, the use of essential oils for a healthier, happier you is easy. While we touched on a few ways essential oils can be used, in the following chapters you'll discover how to get the most out of aromatherapy.

For solo artists (those of you who like to do things on your own), aromatherapy through scent is the way to go. For example, we know that peppermint is good for the digestive system, but did you know that if you smell it you will get quicker relief than if you ingest it? It's true! A 1963 Japanese experiment discovered this result. There are several ways to use scent, and one of the best and most common ways is through a diffuser. So, while opening a bottle of essential oil and taking a big whiff can be of some help, a diffuser emits the scent continually, creating a pleasant, aromatic, healing environment.

However, some benefits are best received through skin application. For instance, ginger oil, known for its bone healing properties, can be applied directly to a small broken appendage like a toe. (Of course, this is in addition to Western therapy, which may include a splint of some sort.) Keep in mind that essential oils are highly concentrated oils. Make sure you carefully read the manufacturer's instructions for proper usage. Very few essential oils should be applied to the skin or ingested at full strength. Most require dilution, and some should not to be used on the skin or ingested at all.

For those who like to share everything with family, friends, and loved ones, massage may be the therapy you are most drawn to. Touch itself is healing and, when coupled with essential oils, massage can be doubly nurturing. When using essential oils during massage, it's important to add it to what's known as a carrier oil. This dilutes the essential oil

somewhat, and makes it go farther. The general rule is to add anywhere from 10-30 drops into an ounce of quality carrier oil.

Inhalation, direct application and massage are among the most common ways to use essential oils, but there are many other ways as well. Some other uses for essential oils include, but aren't limited to, facial tonics, jacuzzis, hot tubs, potpourri, humidifiers, mouthwash, perfume, sitz baths, face and body spray, and in creams and lotions. Once you start using aromatherapy, you'll find that it fits into many different aspects of your lifestyle!

GETTING STARTED

The great thing about essential oils is that they are remarkably safe and easy to use. Plus, they have a wide variety of everyday applications. They can be enjoyed just for their pleasant aromas alone, or used for their therapeutic value. Perhaps the whole spectrum of their soothing and healing properties is what appeals to you. No matter what aspect of aromatherapy attracts you, there are a few simple, yet essential things to know before you get started.

Meet the Aroma Families

While you can most definitely start out with one essential oil and branch out from there, you may want to make yourself a starter kit. This basic kit would include at least one essential oil from each aroma "family," so that you can get more benefits from your personal aromatherapy program. Plus, the advantages of essential oils are often increased when blended with other oils.

There are eight families of aromas; because of their complex chemical make-up, some essential oils can be classified under several families:

Citrus, which includes bergamot, citronella, grapefruit, lemon, lime, orange, and tangerine.

Floral, which includes chamomile, geranium, lavender, neroli, and ylang ylang.

Herbaceous, which includes basil, chamomile, clary sage, hyssop, lavender, and rosemary.

Camphoraceous, which includes camphor, eucalyptus, peppermint, rosemary, and tea tree.

Spicy, which includes allspice, anise seed, cinnamon, clove, ginger, and nutmeg.

Resinous, which includes frankincense and myrrh.

Woody, which includes cedarwood, juniper berry, pine, and sandalwood.

Earthy, which includes patchouli.

Starting with eight essential oils may sound overwhelming. It's perfectly acceptable to begin with less. However, it's a good idea to start with at least two: lavender and eucalyptus are fabulous starter oils because they offer a broad range of health benefits, plus they blend well together.

In choosing your oils, it's important to choose scents that you enjoy. If a scent turns you off, you may not get the full benefit of that particular aroma. Additionally, because the oils are concentrated, they may smell stronger than you first anticipated. This is where blending comes in handy. When compatible essential oils are mixed together, the scent can become more delicate and inviting.

The most important thing to remember is there is no wrong choice in aromatherapy. Choose the oils that make your senses happy, and you'll do just fine.

Basic Aromatic Recipes and Applications

There are many ways to use essential oils. Following are some basic methods of use. The recipes that follow are general. For example, while the bath section suggests using 4-8 drops of essential oil, some essential oils are stronger than others so maybe only 2 drops would be required. Therefore, once you've decided which oil you want to use, consult the essential oil section for more specific guidelines.

Aromatic Baths - Essential oils can be added to bath water just for pleasure alone or for therapeutic value. Either way, a long, luxurious soak in aromatic bath water is a treat for all your senses. The basic rule of thumb is to add 4-8 drops of essential oil to the bath after it's been drawn. Use your hand to be sure and agitate the water so the oil will be well dispersed and not just floating on top, then hop on in.

Foot and Hand Baths - People with arthritis, rheumatism, athlete's foot, and assorted skin problems can benefit from hand or foot baths. Use a bowl or small tub big enough for your appendages. Make sure the water isn't too hot; it must be comfortable enough so that your hands or feet can enjoy generous soak time. Add five to six drops of the appropriate essential oil into the bowl or tub and mix it up with your hand to disperse it. Next, place either your feet or hands in the bowl and soak them for about ten to fifteen minutes. Afterwards, dry skin off completely. For added benefit, add a few drops of the same essential oil to a carrier oil and massage into the skin.

Aromatic Shower - As stated earlier, essential oils used with running water will vaporize the scent. However, a wonderful wake-up treatment using essential oils in a shower makes perfect sense. Choose an invigorating scent, and after washing place 2-3 drops on a clean cloth or sponge and rub it briskly all over your body. If using on your face, rub gently. Rinse as normal.

Sauna - The sauna is a wonderful appliance, and is a wonderful treat for both body and skin. The benefits of a sauna can be increased when an essential oil is added to the mix. Blend just two drops of essential to approximately 600 ml of water and throw it on the heat source. Do not use more than two drops, as more could be overpowering. *Caution: Avoid using sweet-smelling aromas, as they may cause nausea or headache when inhaled in such a tight, closed space. Rose, geranium, and ylang ylang are three to avoid; eucalyptus, lemon, peppermint, and pine are four to use.*

Hot and Cold Compresses - There's nothing quite like a compress to help with muscular pain, sprains, and bruises. They also help to reduce pain and congestion in internal organs. However, it's important to know when to use each.

A cold compress is best for recent injuries (sprains, bruises, swellings, and inflammation), and for headaches, migraines, and fever.

A hot compress is best for old injuries, muscular pain, toothache, menstrual cramps, cystitis, boils and abscesses. Additionally, some people with migraines may prefer a hot compress to a cold one.

To make a hot compress, add a few drops of the appropriate essential oil to a bowl of hot (not boiling) water. Take a clean cloth or bandage and soak it in the mixture. Wring out the excess, and place over the affected area. Repeat as often as needed. A cold compress is made in a similar manner, only using your choice of cold or ice water.

Massage - The basic rule is to add 2-3 drops to 1 ounce of carrier oil, and massage on affected area. However, because some essential oils are stronger than others, consult the essential oil section for specific guidelines.

Steam Inhalations - This is a wonderful way to clear the lungs and sinuses of congestion and infection. Add 2-3 drops of the applicable essential oil to a bowl of steaming hot water. Place your face over the bowl, drape a towel over your head, and breathe normally. Do this for a few minutes, then rest. You can repeat these steps a few times in a row, however discontinue if you feel any discomfort. This particular method directly affects the respiratory tract and the blood supply, therefore you may experience quick relief after this therapy.

Direct Application - Even though essential oils are natural and have a long history of safe use, they are highly concentrated botanical oils, and you should use them with common sense and caution. While experienced aromatherapists and reflexologists often practice neat application, individuals just starting to explore the wonderful world of aromatherapy should exercise caution. Essential oils can be inhaled directly from the bottle, and some like to add a few drops to a handkerchief for convenience.

Gargles and Mouthwashes - Some essential oils have the ability to fight bad breath, reduce the pain of a toothache, and to soothe sore throats. The best way to attack these health challenges is through a gargle or mouthwash. A simple way to make one is to add one drop of the applicable essential oil to two teaspoonfuls of cider vinegar, and add to a glass. Stir well to disperse the oil, then fill the glass with warm water; stir again. Gargle and/or rinse with the mixture. Use twice daily.

Vaporization - Two of the most popular and easy-to-use diffusers are the scent diffuser and the particle diffuser. A common scent diffuser is the "lamp ring" or "light bulb ring", which is made to sit on top of a light bulb and use the heat of the bulb to vaporize the oil's scent into the air. Usually 2-3 drops of oil is all that's needed for a scent diffuser. A particle diffuser is a little more advanced, usually an electronic appliance similar to a humidifier that you add a specified amount of oil to. The oil is then diffused into the air. Scent diffusers only diffuse the aroma of the essential oil into the air, while particle diffusers offer greater therapeutic benefit by actually diffusing oil particles into the air. *Caution: Never, ever place essential oils directly onto a hot light bulb. Never leave any diffuser operating unattended. Always follow manufacturer's instructions.*

These are just a few fun and easy ways to use essential oils. You can also add essential oils to scent-free creams, lotions, shampoos, conditioners, and massage oils. Some people add them to the dishwasher and washing machine, and some even place a drop or two on a washcloth and add it to the dryer. Be creative, and make up your own recipes!

BECOMING AN AROMA PRO

Now that we've covered the history and use of essential oils, it's time to get better acquainted with the oils themselves. The following pages will introduce some of the most beloved and useful oils available today. After reading their descriptions, therapeutic uses, and benefits, you'll be able to decide which ones you want in your aromatherapy home kit.

When choosing oils, think first about what you want the aromatics to do for you. For example, perhaps you lead a stressful lifestyle and crave serenity. A calming oil, like lavender, would be a good choice to begin with. However, that one oil may not be enough, as anyone who leads a stressful lifestyle probably also needs a lot of energy as well. Orange, or any other citrus oil, would be a good one to add to your kit for several reasons. Not only will the citrus oils work to recharge your energy, but they also blend well with lavender. So, as you read over the oils, be sure to check out the "Mixes Well With" section provided for each oil. This will help you make choices that will give your home kit synergy.

Secondly, be sure to get aromatics that you enjoy, otherwise you may not experience their full power. For instance, rose oil is a powerful aromatic, and is great for skin care and emotional balance. However, if you don't like the scent of roses, then your body won't respond as favorably as it would to another oil with a scent you find pleasing. This is true because scent is very subjective, and one reason aromatherapy works is because it builds on what already appeals to and pleases you.

Finally, be sure to read the safety information provided for each oil. While the essential oils listed in this book are perfectly safe for home use, some require special caution, especially if you have been diagnosed with certain medical conditions. Additionally, because essential oils are highly concentrated, it's always a good idea to mix essential oils with a carrier oil before applying on skin. And while some aromatherapists advocate ingesting small amounts of these oils, we do not. Consumption is not necessary in order to receive the full benefits of these oils.

Blending

Many times, you'll find that one oil is all you need to meet a specific need or combat an ailment. However, there will also be times that blending several oils together will offer you a more complete range of benefits to fully address a wide spectrum of needs. You can blend oils on your own, or purchase ready-made blends. Blending is easy and fun. Use your intuition when picking out the oils. Experiment freely, using different oils in different amounts for different effects. Try blending with three oils first, and see how that goes. In most cases, three is all you need for a synergistic blend.

Bergamot, geranium, lavender, and the citrus oils blend well with most of the other oils. However, don't feel confined to having one of these oils in a blend. Some blends that may give you the most benefit won't contain any of these oils at all.

Scintillating Combinations

When combining essential oils, there are no hard and fast rules. A few drops of this, a few drops of that, and a splash of something else and you're set. However, here are some blends that address some common concerns:

Clarity of mind/concentration at work or school: Rosemary, geranium, and basil.

Stress relief: Lavender, lemon, chamomile, myrrh, sandalwood, frankincense, ylang ylang, and cedarwood.

Blues chaser/mood lifter: Orange, eucalyptus, lavender, and neroli.

Pain relief (muscle/joint): Frankincense, ginger, lavender, peppermint, and rosemary.

Colds, cough, and flu: Eucalyptus, ginger, and rosemary.

Wake-up/energy: bergamot, neroli, geranium, and lemon.

The above are just a few examples of useful combinations. Mix together your favorites and make your own personal blends.

Storing

After you've made your own blend, store it in an amber bottle with an airtight seal. If the blend has been mixed with lotions, creams, or ready-made massage oils, the mixture will last only as long as the carrier oil (usually around six months). To make the blend last longer, add wheatgerm oil. It will act as a preservative and extend the shelf life.

Caring for Your Oils

To prolong shelf life and to get the most out of your essential oils, it's important to take a few storage precautions. First and foremost, essential oils are extremely sensitive to light, temperature extremes, and oxygen. To protect the oils from light, make sure they are housed in brown- or amber-colored bottles. Always make sure the lid is on tight, and store in a cool, dark place. Refrigeration is also an option, however be warned that some oils stored this way will become cloudy in nature, but the cloudiness will not affect their therapeutic nature.

Should you choose to store your oils in the refrigerator, take them out an hour before using. When cold, the essential oils don't flow as freely, so letting them warm up a bit naturally will make them easier to use.

The normal shelf life for most essential oils is two years. However, it's possible that with proper care, some may last as long as six years.

One last thing to keep in mind in the care of your oils is this: when blended with lotions, creams, or ready-made massage oils, the essential oil blend will last only about two months. For best results, mix in small amounts, and use up quickly.

Some people prefer to use certified organic essential oils. Organic essential oils are produced from herbs that are grown without the use of synthetic fertilizers and pesticides, irradiation, genetic engineering, growth hormones or antibiotics. They're as close to natural as you can get. Some aromatherapists prefer to use organic essential oils because of their high quality and the fact that they're unadulterated - none of the undesirable substances listed above. While non-organic essential oils labeled 100% pure are usually more than adequate for the casual aromatherapist, some prefer the most natural essential oils possible. Whether you choose 100% pure essential oils or organic essential oils, you can't go wrong. It's really just a matter of preference.

On Your Way
So curl up in your favorite chair with a cup of herbal tea, and get acquainted with the oils. As you read, you'll find yourself drawn to certain ones. Those will be the ones you'll want to include in your starter kit.

Now get started!

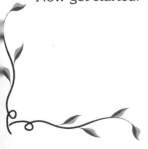

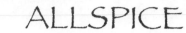

ALLSPICE
(Pimenta diocia)

Many people think that allspice is a combination of several spices, and are surprised to discover it's actually just one. That's because allspice has a flavor reminiscent of a blend of cloves, cinnamon, and nutmeg. Because of its unique flavor, allspice is a favorite of bakers everywhere, and is used in a variety of dishes, from breads, pies, cakes, relishes, gravies, preserves, and even ketchup. Although allspice is highly esteemed for its place in the kitchen, it is also a widely used aromatic as well, with a variety of "scentsational" benefits.

Therapeutic uses: Chest infection, colds, cough, digestive aid, muscle pain, toothache.

Essential Oil Applications:

For chest infection, cold, or cough mix 2-3 drops per ounce of carrier oil and rub into chest and back. Because allspice can irritate skin if used alone, it's important to use it diluted in a carrier oil.

For muscle pain, mix 2-3 drops in once ounce of carrier oil, and rub into affected area.

For toothache, use 2-3 drops on a cotton swab, and apply directly to tooth. Take great care not to swallow, as allspice in this high concentration could cause nausea.

Mixes well with: Geranium, ginger, lavender, orange, myrrh, patchouli, and ylang ylang.

Extraction method: Steam distillation.

Parts used: Leaves and fruit.

Safety Information: Not recommended for use if pregnant. Should not be used neat on skin; always mix with carrier oil, lotion, or cream if using on skin.

FUN FACT:
The ardent explorer Christopher Columbus discovered allspice in 1494, but it wasn't until the 17th century that it was recognized and used as a spice.

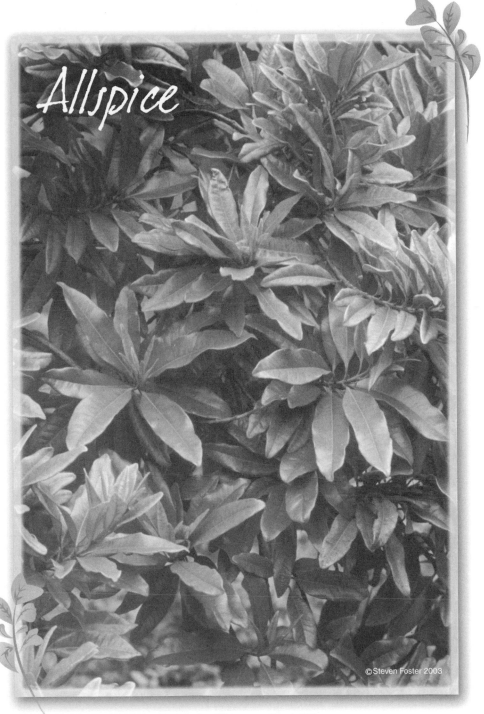

Allspice

©Steven Foster 2003

(See Color Photo on Page 71)

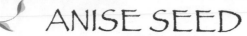

ANISE SEED
(Pimpinella anisum)

From the sublime to the fantastic, Anise Seed has experienced a multitude of uses during the course of history. It was used to perfume the clothing of King Edward IV, as a food flavoring during the Middle Ages, and to fund repairs on the London Bridge, for which a special tax was added to the sale of anise seed. Pliny the Elder, author of the first encyclopedia, claimed its seeds had the power to prevent bad dreams if placed beneath the sleeper's pillow. Anise seed (or aniseed) is a member of the parsley family, and its flavor resembles licorice. Used medicinally since prehistoric times, anise seed remains a staple in aromatherapy.

Therapeutic uses: Asthma, breath freshener, bronchitis, colds, coughs, digestive aid, flatulence, flu, hiccups, menopausal discomforts, migraine, muscle aches, nausea, pleasant dreams, rheumatism, sneezing, stomach cramps, vertigo, whooping cough.

Essential Oil Applications:

For abdominal and stomach cramps, and severe sneezing: mix 5 drops of anise seed oil with 1 tablespoon of almond oil, and massage into stomach (cramps) or neck (sneezing). Use same mixture for coughs, but massage onto chest instead.

For asthma, bronchitis, colds, coughs, flu, and whooping cough, use 2-3 drops in a steam inhalation. Can also be used in a diffuser.

As a digestive aid and to quell hiccups, use 2-3 drops in a steam inhalation.

To freshen breath, mix one to two drops in warm water. Swish and gargle.

For menstrual discomfort or muscle aches, use 2-3 drops in one ounce of carrier oil and massage on affected area.

For migraines or vertigo, use 2-3 drops on a handkerchief and inhale periodically. Also useful for digestive problems.

To alleviate nausea, use 2-3 drops in a steam inhalation.

For pleasant dreams, mix with chamomile and use in a diffuser.

ANISE SEED
(*Pimpinella anisum*)

Mixes well with: Cedarwood, clary sage, lavender, orange, rosewood, sandalwood, and tangerine.

Extraction method: Steam distillation.

Parts used: Seeds.

Safety Information: Not recommended for use if pregnant. May cause stomach irritation and dizziness, so do not exceed recommended dosage. Do not use if diagnosed with endometriosis or estrogen-dependent cancers.

FUN FACT:
In 1619, it was decreed by law from the Virginia Assembly that each family plant at least six anise seeds a year.

(See Color Photo on Page 71)

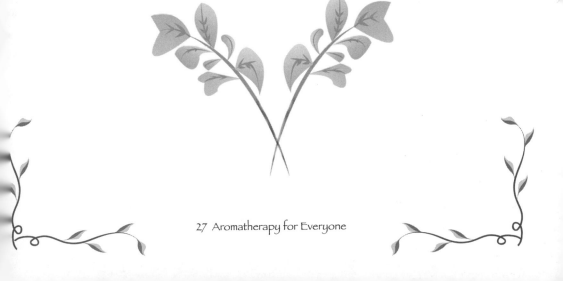

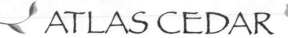

ATLAS CEDAR
(Cedrus atlantica)

Warm, sweet, rich, and woody, the use of cedar oil can be traced back to Biblical times. The Atlas cedar is related to the well-known centuries-old biblical cedars of Lebanon. Today those trees are protected by law from being felled, but the constituents of Atlas cedar oil are very much like its ancestors, and provide many of the same therapeutic benefits. Atlas cedar oil is used in many perfumes and soaps. It produces a calm, meditative state of mind, and has the ability to relieve nervous tension, anger, and stress. When used in a diffuser, Atlas cedar oil can set a calm, quiet atmosphere, perfect for relaxing, meditating, and reflecting. However, its powers aren't restricted to the nervous system; Atlas cedar oil also works wonders on respiratory and immune systems, and is great for skin. Tibetans still use use it in their traditional medicine practices for a variety of ailments.

Therapeutic uses: Acne, aggression, agitation, air purifier, anger, anxiety, arthritis, asthma, bladder disorders, blemishes, bronchitis, cellulite, colds, coughs, cystitis, dandruff, eczema, fluid retention, hair loss, immune system, insect repellent, kidney disorders, meditation, nervous tension, oily hair, oily skin, rheumatism, skin fungus, skin ulcers, stress, vertigo.

Essential Oil Applications:

For arthritis and rheumatism, add 2-3 drops to 1 ounce of carrier oil and massage into affected areas. Can also add 8-10 drops in bath water.

For acne, blemishes, eczema, oily skin, skin fungus or skin ulcers, mix 2-3 drops in 1 ounce of carrier oil and dab on affected areas.

As air purifier, use 2-3 drops in a diffuser.

To alleviate aggression, agitation, anger, anxiety, nervous tension, and vertigo, use 2-3 drops in a diffuser.

For asthma, bronchitis, colds, and coughs, use 2-3 drops in a steam inhalation.

For bladder disorders, cystitis, and kidney disorders, use 8-10 drops in bath water.

ATLAS CEDAR
(Cedrus atlantica)

For cellulite and fluid retention, add 2-3 drops to 1 ounce of carrier oil and massage into affected areas. Can also use 8-10 drops in bath water.

For dandruff or oily scalp, mix 2-3 drops with unscented hair conditioner; massage on scalp. Leave on for 3-5 minutes, then rinse.

To slow hair loss, mix 2-3 drops in 1 ounce of carrier oil and massage on scalp periodically.

To boost the immune system, use 8-10 drops in bath water, or use 2-3 drops in a diffuser.

To repel insects, use a few drops on cotton balls and place in infested areas. Great for ants and moths, but fights against other insects as well.

To keep meditation focused, use 2-3 drops in a diffuser during meditation.

Mixes well with: Bergamot, clary sage, ginger, juniper berry, marjoram, oregano, patchouli, pine, rosemary, rosewood, and ylang ylang.

Extraction method: Steam distillation.

Parts used: Wood, stumps, sawdust.

Safety Information: Avoid if pregnant. Do not use if diagnosed with high blood pressure or heart problems. Possible irritant to skin in sensitive types. Do a patch test first. Because scent is stimulating, it may counteract the sedative effects of drugs like pentobarbital. Do not use consecutively for more than a few days at a time.

> **FUN FACT:**
> The fragrance of cedar was believed to lead worshippers closer to God, consequently many temples were made from it.

(See Color Photo on Page 71)

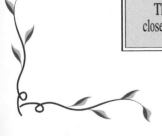

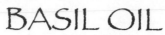

BASIL OIL

(Ocimum basilicum)

Believed by Hindus to be a passport to heaven, and by one Greek author to exist only to drive men insane, basil has had quite the reputation throughout history. However, basil is most associated with food, where it is used as an herb to punch up dishes because of its aromatic, mildly pungent flavor. Basil is a favorite among Italian cooks, and can be found in a variety of native dishes. Though many people associate basil with Italy, it is actually native to India and Iran. In India, basil was considered sacred. In fact, the very name comes from the Greek word *basileus* meaning "king." Currently, there are over 150 varieties of basil, however the variety named *ociumum basilicum* is most used in aromatherapy.

Therapeutic uses: Anti-viral, arthritis, anxiety, colds and flu, concentration, depression, headaches and migraines, menstrual regulation, mental and physical fatigue, muscular spasm, tension, respiratory disorders, rheumatism, stress, weak nervous conditions

Essential Oil Applications:

For anti viral and antibacterial protection, use in a diffuser.

To help alleviate anxiety, depression, mental and physical fatigue, tension, and stress, use 2-3 drops in a diffuser. Can also add 2-3 drops of oil to one ounce of carrier oil and massage on body. For added benefit, add lavender and/or peppermint to the mix.

For arthritis, muscle spasms, or rheumatism, use 2-3 drops in one ounce of carrier oil and massage affected areas. Can also be added to a hot compress.

For congestion, use 2-3 drops of oil in one ounce of carrier oil. Massage on chest and upper back.

To improve concentration, use 2-3 drops in a diffuser.

For headaches or migraines, use 2-3 drops in a hot or cold compress (whichever works best for you).

To help regulate menstrual cycle, use 2-3 drops in a diffuser regularly.

BASIL OIL
(Ocimum basilicum)

For respiratory disorders, use 2-3 drops in a steam inhalation.

Mixes well with: Camphor, citronella, citrus oils, clove, eucalyptus, geranium, lavender, myrrh, oregano, peppermint, rosemary, sandalwood, spearmint, and tea tree.

Extraction method: Steam distillation.

Parts used: Leaves and flowering tops.

Safety Information: Avoid if pregnant. Can irritate skin, therefore do not use without diluting. Use a patch test before using on skin.

FUN FACT:
In Italy, basil is regarded as a sign of love.

(See Color Photo on Page 71)

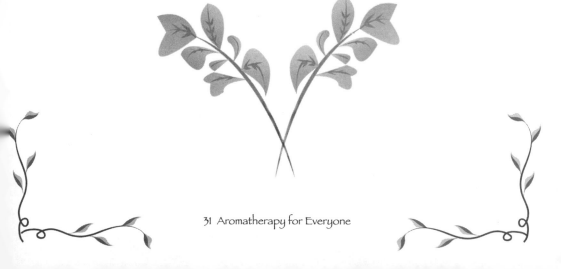

BERGAMOT
(Citrus bergamia)

Bergamot has a rather controversial history. Some say it originates from Northern Italy, taking its name from the the small town of Bergamo where it was discovered. Others state it originated in India, and its Turkish name means "King of Pears", which reflects the pear-shaped fruit of the plant. Whatever it's history, there is no disputing that bergamot has been used for years because of its sweet, citrusy scent with spicy undertones. Popular with perfumers for centuries, bergamot has an uplifting, energizing scent which also makes it perfect for aromatherapy. Additionally, bergamot is one of the most versatile essential oils, as not only does it have sedative qualities, but also stimulating as well. It appears to adapt to the needs of the person using it. Bergamot also gives Earl Grey tea its unmistakable and unique flavor, which makes it a favorite among tea lovers everywhere.

Therapeutic uses: Acne, appetite regularity, anxiety, colds and flu, cystitis, depression, digestive system, eczema, fatigue, fever, flatulence, halitosis, infection (all types, especially skin), mouth infections, nervous tension, sore throat, stress, tonsillitis, urinary tract.

Essential Oil Applications:

For acne, eczema, psoriasis, and wounds, mix 2-3 drops with jojoba carrier oil and apply directly to affected area.

To alleviate anxiety, depression, fatigue, nervous tension, and stress use 2-3 drops of essential oil in a diffuser or a lamp ring.

For cystitis and urinary tract health, use 4-5 drops in bath water for a luxurious, long soak. Also, 2-3 drops of bergamot can be added to a carrier oil and massaged over the lower abdomen and kidney area to promote optimal health of the excretory system.

For digestive help and flatulence, use 2-3 drops in a carrier oil and massage over abdomen area. Can also use 2-3 drops in a diffuser.

For halitosis, mouth infections, sore throat, or tonsillitis, use 2-3 drops in a homemade mouthwash. Gargle and rinse.

To regulate appetite, use 2-3 drops in a diffuser regularly.

BERGAMOT
(Citrus bergamia)

Mixes well with: All essential oils, and especially Atlas cedarwood, citronella, chamomile, clary sage, eucalyptus, geranium, juniper, lavender, lemon, lime, marjoram, nutmeg, orange, oregano, palmarosa, rosemary, sandalwood, tangerine, and ylang ylang.

Extraction method: Cold expression

Parts used: Peel of nearly ripe fruit.

Safety Information: This essential oil is phytotoxic, which means it increases the effect of sunlight. Therefore, never apply bergamot to skin before exposure to sun. Additionally, do not apply neat on skin; must be diluted in a carrier oil or cream. Not recommended for use if pregnant.

FUN FACT:
Bergamot essence is used in voodoo as a protective measure against evil and danger.

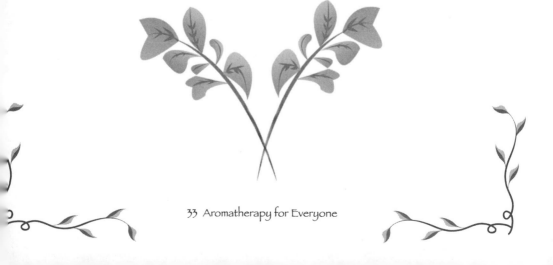

CAMPHOR
(Cinnamomum camphora)

Powerful and medicinal are two words to describe the unique scent of camphor. Because of its strong aroma, peasants used to wear lumps of camphor around their necks to repel infectious diseases. For over 5,000 years Ayurvedic medicine has utilized camphor mainly as a germ killer. Camphor was also used in Persia (now Iran) as a remedy for the plague. Even modern day people turn to camphor to fight cold symptoms. Besides fighting colds, camphor has many other uses. Ancient inhabitants of India used camphor in a variety of religious rituals. The Chinese used camphor wood to build ships and temples, not just for the wood's durability, but also because of its aromatic properties. Camphor has another unique use: that of a moth repellent. Therefore, it's a great natural way to protect much-loved wardrobes from the damage moth infestation causes.

Therapeutic uses: Bronchitis, bruises, chills, colds and flu, coughs, insect repellent, muscle pain, sprains.

Essential Oil Applications:

For bronchitis, colds and flu, and coughs place 2-3 drops in a diffuser or lamp ring.

To repel insects, place 2-3 drops in a diffuser or lamp ring. Can also be used on cotton and placed in closet, however do not place directly on clothes.

For bruises, muscle pain, and sprains use in a cold compress.

Great as an after-sun tonic, however do not use directly on skin. Mix a couple of drops in two-three tablespoons of liquid lanolin and apply to skin. Do a patch test first to check for sensitivity.

Mixes well with: Basil, chamomile, lavender.

Safety Information: Camphor is one of the strongest essential oils available, therefore caution must be exercised when using this particular oil. Do not use if pregnant or nursing, or if diagnosed with epilepsy or asthma. Do not take internally.

FUN FACT:
Camphor is used in some cultures to scare away ghosts.

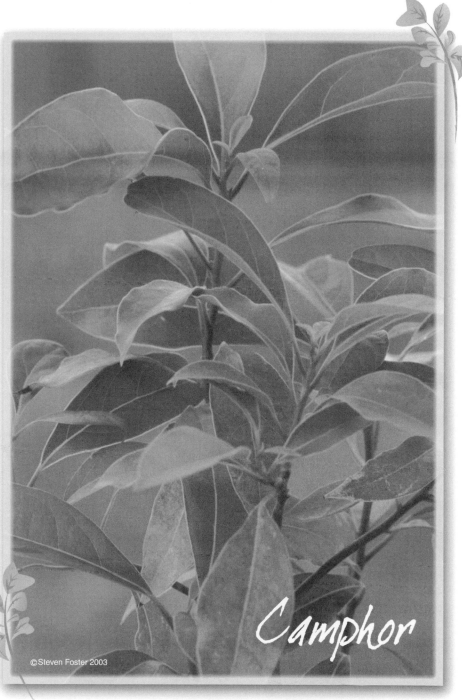

© Steven Foster 2003

Camphor

(See Color Photo on Page 71)

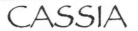

CASSIA

(Cinnamomum cassia)

Cassia, also known as Chinese cinnamon, is somewhat similar to cinnamon *(Cinnamomum zeylanicum)* in both taste and therapeutic properties. Although the United States Pharmacopoeia recognizes it as cinnamon, it should not be confused as such, for it has it's own unique benefits and history. It has been used for centuries both medicinally and culinarily. Germans and Romans preferred to use cassia instead of cinnamon in chocolate, as it has a stronger flavor. Both Europeans and Chinese used cassia in a variety of ways to spice up foods. The Chinese also use cassia frequently for digestive complaints like diarrhea and nausea. It's also used to fight colds, rheumatism, kidney and reproductive complaints, and most particularly vascular disorders. Cassia is also a known skin irritant, so it's best to use it in vapor therapy. Today, cassia is often used in confectionaries and potpourri.

Therapeutic uses: Arthritis, colds, diarrhea, germicide, kidney problems, nausea, reproductive complaints, rheumatism, vascular disorders.

Essential Oil Applications:

For arthritis, colds, diarrhea, kidney problems, nausea, reproductive complaints, rheumatism, and vascular disorders, use 2-3 drops in a diffuser.

As a powerful germicide, cassia oil can be mixed with water and sprayed in a sick room.

Mixes well with: Cassia is best used on its own.

Extraction method: Steam or water distillation.

Parts used: Leaves (steam), or bark, leaves, twigs and stalks (water).

Safety Information: Avoid if pregnant. Very large doses can cause depression.

FUN FACT:
In the Middle Ages, Europeans used dried cassia buds
in Hippocras, a spiced wine.

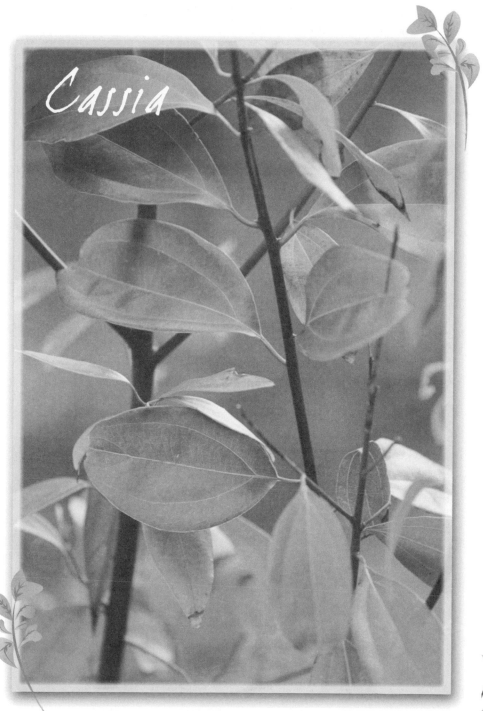

Cassia

(See Color Photo on Page 71)

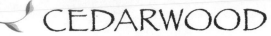

CEDARWOOD

(Juniperus virginiana)

If the smell of a newly sharpened pencil brings back good memories, you'll love the mild, sweet, woody scent of cedarwood. Native Americans valued cedarwood for its healing and purification properties. They used it to combat respiratory infections, and also to treat arthritis, skin rashes, and kidney infections. Cedarwood was also used in some ceremonies for purification. Egyptians also embraced cedarwood, and used it in the mummification process, cosmetics, and to repel insects. Insects and rats hate the smell of cedarwood, therefore it makes a great repellent, especially against mosquitoes, moths, and woodworms. In fact, at one time cedarwood was combined with citronella and used as a commercial insecticide. Today, aromatherapists use cedarwood in a variety of capacities, from insect repellent to mood relaxer.

Therapeutic uses: Acne, arthritis, asthma, bronchitis, congestion, coughs, cystitis, dandruff, eczema, insect repellent, kidney disorders, nervous tension, oily skin, psoriasis, rheumatism, stress-related disorders, and urinary tract infections.

Essential Oil Applications:

For arthritis and rheumatism, add 2-3 drops to 1 ounce of carrier oil and massage into affected areas. Can also add 8-10 drops in bath water.

For acne, eczema, psoriasis, and oily skin, mix 2-3 drops in 1 ounce of carrier oil and dab on affected areas.

For asthma, bronchitis, congestion, and coughs, use 2-3 drops in a steam inhalation.

To alleviate nervous tension and stress-related disorders, use 2-3 drops in a diffuser.

For cystitis, kidney disorders, or urinary tract infections, use 8-10 drops in bath water.

For dandruff, mix 2-3 drops with unscented hair conditioner; massage on scalp. Leave on for 3-5 minutes, then rinse.

To repel insects and rats, use a few drops on cotton balls and place in infested areas. Can also use 2-3 drops in a diffuser.

CEDARWOOD
(Juniperus virginiana)

Mixes well with: Anise, bergamot, citronella, chamomile, eucalyptus, ginger, juniper berry, lavender, lemon, palmarosa, patchouli, pine, rosemary, and sandalwood.

Extraction method: Steam distillation.

Parts used: Wood chips and sawdust.

Safety Information: Avoid if pregnant. Possible irritant to skin in sensitive types. Do a patch test first.

FUN FACT:
Cedarwood is used to make pencils, which makes its aroma reminiscent of school days gone by.

(See Color Photo on Page 72)

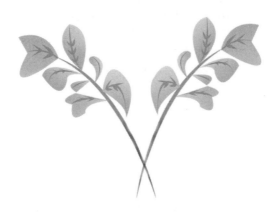

MAROC CHAMOMILE
(Ormenis multicaulis)

Chamomile is the great relaxer. It's been used for centuries to calm and soothe the mind, body, and soul. In fact, in the language of flowers its name means "patience in adversity." Maroc chamomile *(Ormenis multicaulis)* should not be confused with German or Roman chamomiles as it has it's own set of unique benefits. This particular chamomile is good for ailments such as sensitive skin, colic, colitis, headache and migraine, irritability, insomnia, and menopause. While effective on its own, chamomile can help boost the power of lavender and cedarwood essential oils.

Therapeutic uses: Colic, colitis, headache and migraine, irritability, insomnia, liver and spleen congestion, menopause, sensitive skin.

Essential Oil Applications:

For colic, colitis, and liver or spleen congestion, add 5-8 drops to one ounce of carrier oil and massage on body. Can also add 8-10 drops to bath water or a few drops to a diffuser.

For headache or migraine, use 2-3 drops in a hot or cold compress (whichever works best for you).

For insomnia, use 5-6 drops in a diffuser. Can also place 2-3 drops on a tissue, and place inside your pillow before bedtime. Replace nightly. For added benefit, add lavender to the mix.

To help lessen the effects of menopause on the body, add 8 drops to one ounce of carrier oil and massage on body regularly. Can also add a few drops to a diffuser nightly, and 8-10 drops to bath water.

For sensitive skin, dilute one drop of chamomile with 1 teaspoon of a carrier oil, like sweet almond, and dab on skin.

Mixes well with: Cedarwood and lavender.

Extraction method: Steam distillation

MAROC CHAMOMILE
(Ormenis multicaulis)

Parts used: Flowering tops.

Safety Information: Generally safe, however it is best to avoid if pregnant.

FUN FACT:
Before chemical hair dye became widely available, chamomile was traditionally used to lighten hair.

(See Color Photo on Page 72)

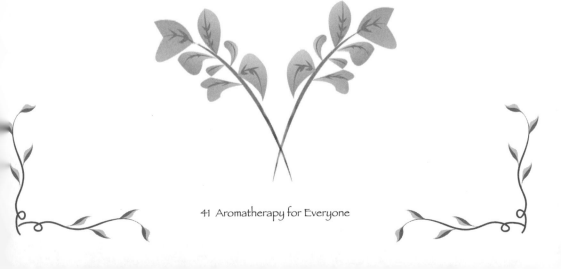

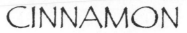

CINNAMON
(Cinnamomum zeylanicum)

The smell of cinnamon wafting through the kitchen is probably the most beloved aroma of the Earth's population. First mentioned in Chinese literature as early as 2700 BC, cinnamon is considered a "warm" herb and is valued in many ancient traditional medical systems, including Ayurvedic medicine. Early Europeans considered cinnamon a "rare and precious spice", and it was often used in tonics to treat coughs, colds and digestive ailments. Used in just about every kitchen of every culture, cinnamon is treasured for its culinary magic as well as its therapeutic benefits. However, the kitchen and the doctor's office aren't the only places this delicious spice shines. It is also highly valued in the world of aromatherapy for its warming and comforting qualities. Cinnamon is especially good for colds, flu, arthritis, rheumatism, and other aches and pains. It also blends well other oils, especially citrus and spice scents. Cinnamon oil is also great to use in a diffuser before parties or open houses, as it lends a homey, welcoming quality people find comforting and appealing.

Therapeutic uses: Arthritis, bronchitis, chills, colds, diarrhea, flu, intestinal infections, libido, menstrual pain, nervous exhaustion, poor circulation, rheumatism, sluggish digestion, sneezing, stress-related conditions.

Essential Oil Applications:

Because cinnamon oil should never be used in bath or neat on skin, vapor therapy is most recommended for the above ailments. Use 2-5 drops in a diffuser. For severe respiratory conditions, like acute bronchitis, steam inhalation is also a viable alternative. Can also add 3-4 drops to 1 ounce of carrier oil and massage on body, however this is not recommended for those with sensitive skin.

Mixes well with: Bergamot, clove, frankincense, geranium, ginger, grapefruit, lavender, lemon, marjoram, nutmeg, orange, patchouli, rose, rosemary, tangerine, thyme, and ylang ylang.

Extraction method: Steam distillation.

CINNAMON
(Cinnamomum zeylanicum)

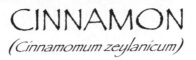

Parts used: Leaves and twigs (dried inner bark).

Safety Information: Avoid if pregnant. Not to be used if under age 18. People with sensitive skin should avoid cinnamon completely. Do not use in baths. Can irritate mucous membranes, so use with care.

FUN FACT:
Cinnamon was once so highly valued that it was used as a trade commodity between India, China and Egypt.

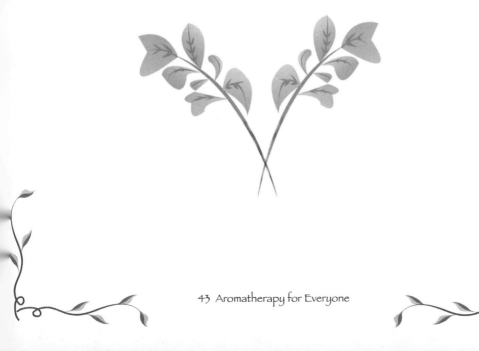

CITRONELLA
(Cymbopogon winterianus)

Citronella is a scent every one knows, but might not love. It's so strong that even insects are affected by its scent. Used for centuries mainly as an insect repellent, citronella actually has a wide variety of other uses. Look closely, and you'll find it as an ingredient in many perfumes, soaps, skin lotions, and deodorants. Citronella is a versatile essential oil, and is a must for anyone who lives in a hot, humid environment.

Therapeutic uses: digestive complaints, excessive perspiration, fatigue, feline repellent, fleas, headache, insect repellent, migraine, oily skin, sickroom freshener.

Essential Oil Applications:

For dogs with fleas, add a couple of drops to a "doggie bandana" or to an absorbent collar, such as woven nylon, and place around dog's neck. *Do not use this method for cats, as felines are much more sensitive to this scent.*

For digestive complaints, mix 2 drops with 2-3 tablespoons of a carrier oil and massage on abdominal area.

For headaches and migraines, use 2-3 drops in a cold or hot compress.

As an insect repellent, use a few drops in a burner, vaporizer, or diffuser. Works especially well if used by an open window. Be careful if used indoors, as it can adversely affect caged birds.

As a moth repellent, place a few drops on a cotton ball, and place in closet or linen closet. Refresh periodically.

For oily skin, mix 2-3 drops with a carrier oil, and dab on face with a cotton ball.

To keep neighborhood cats from digging up your garden, mix 10-12 drops of oil in a plastic spray bottle full of water, and spray around your garden. Do not spray directly on plants.

CITRONELLA
(Cymbopogon winterianus)

As a deodorant, mix 2-3 drops with a carrier oil and apply to arm pits.

For those who are bedridden, citronella is a great freshener for the "sickroom." Place a couple of drops in a diffuser or lamp ring. Will also help to clear the mind at the same time.

Mixes well with: Basil, bergamot, cedarwood, eucalyptus, geranium, lavender, lemon, lime, oregano, pennyroyal, pine, rosemary, orange, and tea tree.

Extraction method: Steam distillation.

Parts Used: Fresh, part-dried, or dried grass.

Safety Information: Do not use while pregnant.

FUN FACT:
Citronella has been used in exorcism rituals to get rid of demons.

(See Color Photo on Page 72)

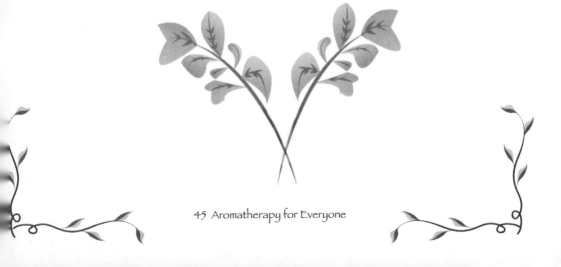

CLARY SAGE
(Salvia sclarea)

Clary Sage was highly valued during the Middle Ages for its ability to to heal all sorts of eye problems. Called "clarus", meaning clear, it was later transformed into clary. Part of its Latin name, salvia, means to save. Rightly so, as clary sage enjoys a reputation as a sort of "cure all" because it quite literally is used successfully to restore health in a variety of areas. Egyptians loved clary sage for its purported ability to cure infertility. The Greeks, Romans, and Chinese loved it because it held promise to assure long life. And 16th century Englanders loved it as a replacement for hops to brew beer. Clary sage is also a favorite of creative types, who swear that its fragrance is inspirational. Why not open a bottle yourself and take a whiff? Maybe clary sage will inspire you to greatness!

Therapeutic uses: Anxiety, back pain, decreased libido, depression, digestive disorders, insomnia, inflammation, menopause, neck strain, nervous tension, muscle pain, premenstrual syndrome, respiratory health, skin problems, stress.

Essential Oil Applications:

For anxiety, decreased libido, depression, insomnia, menopause, nervous tension, and stress use 2-3 drops as a vapor therapy, or use in a diffuser or lamp ring. Can also add 2-3 drops to a carrier oil and massage on body.

For back pain, neck strain, and skin problems, mix 2-3 drops of oil with 2-3 tablespoons of liquid lanolin and apply to problem areas for relief.

For discomfort associated with menopause or premenstrual syndrome, use 4-5 drops in bath water for a relaxing soak. You can also use 2-3 drops on a handkerchief and inhale during time of discomfort. However, do not inhale for long periods of time, as prolonged exposure could cause a headache.

For respiratory problems, place 2-3 drops of oil in a diffuser or lamp ring.

CLARY SAGE
(Salvia sclarea)

Mixes well with: Anise, bergamot, cedarwood, citrus oils, clove, frankincense, geranium, grapefruit, hyssop, jasmine, juniper, lavender, lime, marjoram, nutmeg, palmarosa, patchouli, pine, rose, tangerine, tea tree, and thyme.

Extraction method: Steam distillation.

Parts used: Flowering tops.

Safety Information: Avoid during pregnancy. Long periods of inhalation could cause headaches. Alcohol consumption while using clary sage could increase the effects of alcohol, so it's wise not to imbibe during use.

> ## FUN FACT:
> Centuries ago, German winemakers added clary sage to inferior wines to make them more intoxicating.

(See Color Photo on Page 72)

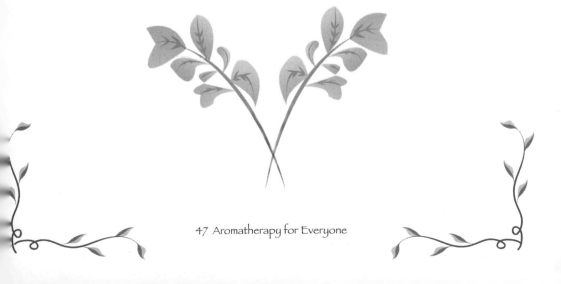

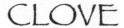

CLOVE
(Eugenia caryophyllata)

Cloves were important in the earliest spice trades, probably because of their importance in flavoring foods. Known for their hot, spicy, pungent flavor, cloves are a favorite seasoning spice for meats, baked goods, and beverages. Besides its beloved place in the kitchen, clove essential oil is a valued aromatic, and used traditionally as a remedy for skin conditions, to calm digestive upset, and to relieve nausea. However, it's best known for its use as both a breath freshener and toothache reliever. Cloves remain an important spice commodity, and today are used in everything from perfume to mulled wines and from love potions to pomades.

Therapeutic uses: Airborne bacteria, arthritis, asthma, bad breath, bronchitis, burns and cuts, chest infections, colds and chills, diarrhea, exhaustion, flu, mental debility, muscle pain or spasms, nausea, toothache, rheumatism, stress, tired limbs, warts.

Essential Oil Applications:

To fight against airborne bacteria, use 2-3 drops in a diffuser.

For arthritis, muscle spasms, and rheumatism, add 1 drop to 1 ounce of carrier oil and massage on affected areas.

For asthma, bronchitis, chest infections, and other respiratory problems, use 2-3 drops in a steam inhalation. Can also use a few drops in a diffuser.

For burns, cuts, and warts, mix 2-3 drops to 1 ounce of carrier oil and dab on affected area.

For colds, chills, and flu, add 2-3 drops to 1 ounce of carrier oil and massage on chest.

To help with diarrhea, use 2-3 drops in 1 ounce of carrier oil and massage on lower back and abdomen.

To help alleviate exhaustion, stress, and to strengthen mental function, add 2-3 drops in a diffuser. Can also add 2-3 drops to 1 ounce of carrier oil and massage on body.

CLOVE
(Eugenia caryophyllata)

As a mouthwash to help knock out bad breath, dilute in water or clear alcohol (1% clove oil). Swish in mouth, spit out, and rinse with water.

For toothache, put 2-3 drops on a cotton swab and place directly on tooth. Can also add 1 drop to 1 ounce of carrier oil, and massage into jawline.

Mixes well with: Cinnamon, clary sage, geranium, ginger, grapefruit, jasmine, lavender, lemon, myrrh, nutmeg, orange, palmarosa, rose, sandalwood, tangerine, tea tree, and ylang ylang.

Extraction method: Steam distillation.

Parts used: Sun-dried buds.

Safety Information: Avoid during pregnancy. Can irritate skin, so make sure to always dilute clove essential oil with a carrier oil, cream, or lotion. Can irritate mucous membranes, so when using a vaporizer or in a diffuser be sure to limit exposure. Do not use on a tooth that is currently being worked on by a dentist for root canal. Do not use in baths.

FUN FACT:
During the Han dynasty, cloves were known as "tongue spice" and courtiers were required to hold cloves in their mouths when talking to the emperor.

(See Color Photo on Page 72)

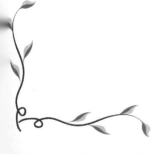

EUCALYPTUS
(Eucalyptus globulus)

Centuries ago, the eucalyptus tree was thought to cleanse the environment, so the frail and sickly would choose to live in areas where these fragrant trees grew, hoping for recovery from their ailments. While just living under the trees might not be the cure people hoped for, the tree does indeed offer healing. The Australian Aborigines applied crushed eucalyptus leaves to wounds to promote healing. They also used eucalyptus leaves to fight infection and relieve muscular pain. In India, eucalyptus is used to cool fever and fight contagious diseases. Even Western surgeons recognized the benefits of eucalyptus, and have used a eucalyptus solution to wash out operation cavities. Today, eucalyptus is used in many different types of pharmaceutical products, from vapor rubs to cold remedies. Even veterinarians and dentists use eucalyptus in their practices. Its sweet, menthol, woody scent coupled with its proven healing abilities makes it a favorite essential oil in aromatherapy.

Therapeutic uses: Antibacterial, asthma, arthritis, chicken pox, coughs, decongestant, fever, insect repellent, measles, migraine, muscle pain, rheumatism, shingles, sinusitis, sprains, throat infections.

Essential Oil Applications:

For arthritis, muscle pains, and rheumatism, mix 2-3 drops in 1 ounce of carrier oil and massage on affected area.

For asthma, coughs, sinusitis, stuffed up noses, and throat infections, use 5-7 drops in a vaporizer. Can also be mixed in a carrier oil and massaged on chest.

To kill airborne bacteria in a sickroom, use in a spray bottle. Mix 10 drops of oil in 1 quart of water; shake well before spraying.

To guard against fly infestation, put droplets of oil on ribbon, and hang near windows or place on windowsills. Refresh weekly.

For chicken pox and shingles, use 2-3 drops on a cotton swab and apply to affected areas. Relieves pain associated with these ailments.

As an insect repellent, mix equal amounts with bergamot and lavender. If applying to skin, use in a carrier oil. If using in a linen closet, apply to cotton balls and place on shelves.

EUCALYPTUS
(Eucalyptus globulus)

To freshen up garbage bins, place a few drops of oil on a paper towel, and wipe over lid or place in the bottom of the bin to both kill germs and smells.

Mixes well with: Basil, bergamot, cedarwood, citronella, ginger, grapefruit, juniper, lavender, lemon, lime, marjoram, orange, oregano, peppermint, pine, rosemary, spearmint, tea tree, and thyme.

Extraction method: Steam distillation.

Parts used: Fresh or partially dried leaves and young twigs.

Safety Information: Avoid during pregnancy. Do not use if diagnosed with high blood pressure or epilepsy. Always use in dilution. Avoid if taking homeopathic remedies, as eucalyptus acts as an antidote against such therapies.

FUN FACT:

In the 19th century, eucalyptus trees were called "fever trees," because they destroyed the breeding ground of the malaria mosquito. The tree grows fast, and uses up large amounts of water, thus large amounts of the trees can turn swamp into usable land – and also rid the area of mosquitos in the process.

(See Color Photo on Page 72)

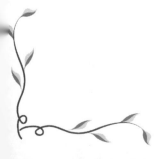
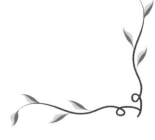

FRANKINCENSE
(Boswellia carteri)

Frankincense was one of the gifts given to the baby Jesus from the three Magi. People often wonder why this is so, after all, isn't it just a nicely scented tree? Actually, at one time, frankincense was valued as highly as gold. It was held in this high regard for thousands of years. Frankincense not only had many healing properties, but was also burned to rid the sick of evil spirits, and to purify body and soul. Because of its ability to slow down and deepen the breath, frankincense helps to keep prayer and meditation focused. Unsurprisingly, the Egyptians used it in the embalming process, but surprisingly they used it in cosmetic face masks as well. Today, frankincense is as highly valued by aromatherapists as it was in days of yore. With benefits that take care of both external and internal problems, it truly is worth its weight in gold.

Therapeutic uses: Aging skin, asthma, bedsores, blemishes, bronchitis, chilliness, colds, coughs, cystitis, fatigue, flu, heavy periods, hemorrhoids, labor, laryngitis, meditation, menstrual health, nasal congestion, oily skin, poor circulation, prayer, respiration, rheumatism, scars, shortness of breath, sores, urinary tract infections, wounds.

Essential Oil Applications:

For asthma, bronchitis, coughs, colds, flu, and laryngitis, use 2-3 drops in 1 ounce of carrier oil. Rub on chest for asthma, bronchitis, coughs, and cold, and on throat for laryngitis. Can also use 2-3 drops in a diffuser or steam inhalation.

For bedsores, scars, and wounds, use 2-3 drops in a cold compress and apply to affected area. Can also be added to a cotton ball and dabbed on directly; use lightly.

For blemishes or oily skin, wet a cotton ball and add a drop or two of oil. Dab affected areas lightly.

To improve circulation, mix 4-5 drops with 1 ounce of carrier oil and massage on body. Can also use in bath water.

To help alleviate fatigue, use 3-5 drops in a diffuser.

For hemorrhoids, add 2-3 drops to 2 tablespoons of liquid lanolin, and massage into affected areas.

During labor, use a few drops in a diffuser. It will help calm the

FRANKINCENSE
(Boswellia carteri)

mother-to-be, and also help her to focus, especially if using Lamaze.

To rejuvenate mature complexions, wash face, then use 2-3 drops with 1 ounce of almond carrier oil, and rub gently onto face.

During menstruation, use 8-10 drops in bath water, and take a nice, long soak. Helps with a variety of menstrual issues, like cramps, loss of focus, and fatigue.

For nasal congestion, sprinkle a few drops on a handkerchief and inhale periodically. Can also add 2-3 drops to a diffuser or steam inhalation.

To help regulate heavy periods, use 3-4 drops in 1 ounce of carrier oil and massage on lower abdomen area regularly.

To help facilitate prayer and/or meditation, use 4-5 drops in a diffuser.

For rheumatism, use 3-5 drops in 1 ounce of carrier oil and massage on affected areas. Can also use in a hot compress.

To help relieve shortness of breath, use 3-5 drops in a steam inhalation or diffuser.

To help alleviate urinary tract infections, use 8-10 drops in bath water, in addition to using doctor prescribed medication.

Mixes well with: Bergamot, cinnamon, clary sage, geranium, grapefruit, jasmine, lavender, lemon, myrrh, neroli, orange, patchouli, pine, rose, sandalwood, tangerine, and ylang ylang.

Extraction method: Steam distillation.

Parts used: Oleoresin.

Safety Information: No special precautions with frankincense, however it's best to use it in moderation.

> ### FUN FACT:
> Frankincense can grow without soil.

(See Color Photo on Page 73)

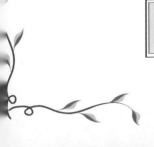

GERANIUM
(Pelargonium graveolens)

Known as the "women's oil" because of its menstrual and menopausal benefits, geranium oil actually has a wide variety of uses. Besides promoting women's health, it's also useful for skin problems, like eczema and athlete's foot, and for respiratory tract health. Its spicy, exotic, floral scent also makes it a fabulous aphrodisiac. Additionally, geranium oil is very gentle, and can be used by almost everybody, anywhere, anytime.

Therapeutic uses: Aphrodisiac, circulatory system health, cold sores, cellulite, digestive mucous, frostbite, headaches, premenstrual syndrome, menopause, mood balancer, mosquito repellent, nervous tension, skin problems (like acne, athlete's foot, and eczema), sore throat, stress and stress-related problems, respiratory system, tonsillitis.

Essential Oil Applications:

For cold sores, place 1 drop on a cotton swab and dab affected area.

For frostbite, massage area with approximately 5 drops of oil.

To balance mood, place 2-3 drops in a diffuser, or place on a cotton ball or handkerchief and inhale deeply 2-3 times.

A bath made with 8-10 drops of oil will help relieve headache, premenstrual syndrome, stress, and tension.

For cellulite, premenstrual syndrome, and menopause, mix 20 drops in 1 ounce of carrier oil and massage on body. For cellulite, massage on affected areas. For premenstrual syndrome and menopause, massage on abdomen and back, paying extra attention to the lower back region.

As a mosquito repellent, use 5 drops in a diffuser. Can also be mixed with citronella for a stronger repellent.

For stress and tension that interferes with a good night's rest, place 4 drops on tissue or cotton ball and place inside pillow case.

GERANIUM
(Pelargonium graveolens)

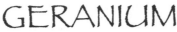

...blems (i.e. acne, athlete's foot, chillblains, dandruff, ... put 2-3 drops on a cotton ball and dab affected area.

To help relieve stress and tension, use 2-3 drops in a diffuser or lamp ring. Can also use 2-3 drops in 1 ounce of carrier oil for a relaxing massage.

For respiratory problems, use 5 drops in a vaporizer.

To relieve a sore throat and to help fight tonsillitis, use 2-5 drops in a steam inhalation.

As an aphrodisiac, use 8-10 drops of oil in a bath or use 2-3 drops in a diffuser or lamp ring.

Mixes well with: Allspice, basil, bergamot, cinnamon, citronella, clary sage, clove, frankincense, ginger, grapefruit, hyssop, jasmine, juniper, lavender, lemon, lime, myrrh, neroli, nutmeg, orange, palmarosa, patchouli, pennyroyal, peppermint, rose, rosemary, rosewood, sandalwood, tangerine, tea tree, thyme, and ylang ylang.

Extraction method: Steam distillation

Parts used: Leaves, stalks, and flowers.

Safety Information: Geranium oil is perfectly safe for home use in moderation. In very large quantities, it may cause irritation to sensitive skin.

FUN FACT:
Geraniums used to be planted outside houses to keep evil spirits away.

(See Color Photo on Page 73)

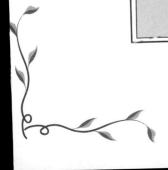

GINGER
(Zingiber officianale)

Though ugly in its natural appearance, ginger is one of the most highly valued spices in the world. Not only does it give food a unique spicy, peppery flavor, it's also renowned for its healing properties. For centuries, different cultures worldwide have embraced it and sung its praises. Traditional Chinese medicine employed the use of fresh ginger for a variety of health issues, from respiratory challenges to toothaches. The Greeks used it to counteract the effects of poison. King Henry VIII of England recommended the use of ginger to combat the the great plague of the 16th century. These days, aromatherapists use its warming and soothing qualities to combat digestive and joint complaints, mood swings, and to help increase libido.

Therapeutic uses: arthritis, backache, chills, circulatory health, cold and flu, decongestant, digestive system, disconnectiveness, fractures, libido, lymphatic system, mood swings, muscle pain, rheumatism, runny nose, sinusitis, sore throat.

Essential Oil Applications:

For mood swings, a general feeling of disconnectiveness, and to shake off the tendency to procrastinate, use 2-3 drops in a diffuser or place on a cotton ball and inhale 2-3 times. This will help to re-energize and revitalize mind, body, and soul.

For arthritis, backache, fractures, muscle pain, and rheumatism, use 2-3 drops in 1 ounce of carrier oil and massage into affected areas. Another choice would be to use 2-3 drops in a hot or cold compress on affected areas.

To stimulate the circulatory system, use 2-3 drops in 1 ounce of carrier oil and massage into body.

For runny nose, sore throat, sinusitis, or as a decongestant use 2-3 drops as a steam inhalation.

To stimulate the lymphatic system, put a couple of drops on a cotton ball, and dab on the arm pit area.

GINGER
(Zingiber officianale)

To revitalize libido, use 2-3 drops in 1 ounce of carrier oil and use as a massage, or diffuse 2-3 drops into air.

Mixes well with: Allspice, Atlas cedarwood, cedarwood, cinnamon, clove, eucalyptus, geranium, grapefruit, jasmine, juniper, lemon, lime, myrrh, orange, palmarosa, patchouli, rose, rosemary, sandalwood, spearmint, tangerine, tea tree, and ylang ylang.

Extraction method: Steam distillation

Part used: Unpeeled, dried, ground root.

Safety Information: Although it is frequently administered to pregnant women to help alleviate morning sickness, it is best to avoid the use of ginger during pregnancy in aromatherapy practices. For people with extremely sensitive skin, dilute oil carefully before using in massage or bath.

FUN FACT:
To rev up their husbands' libidos, the women of Senegal weave ginger root into their belts.

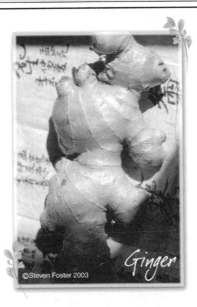

Ginger

©Steven Foster 2003

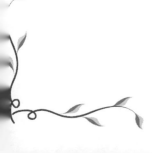
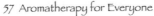
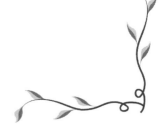

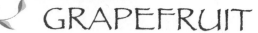

GRAPEFRUIT
(Citrus paradisi)

Grapefruit is a bit of a botanical mystery. It appears to be the hybrid of a sour fruit known as a shaddock and a sweet orange. However, there are no existing records to show that there was a deliberate hybridization of the two plants. So it remains a mystery as to whether it was deliberately bred or was a product of Nature's own type of natural hybridization. First cultivated in the West Indies back in the 18th century, the United States is now the world's largest producer of grapefruit anywhere. Therapeutically, grapefruit has energizing and cleansing properties, plus has a unique ability to aid fat dissolution.

Therapeutic uses: Acne, antiseptic, arthritis, cellulite, depression, detoxification, disinfectant, fluid retention, headaches, mental or nervous exhaustion, menstruation, menstrual cramps, muscle fatigue, rheumatism, stiffness, stress.

Essential Oil Applications:

For arthritis, muscle fatigue, rheumatism, and stiffness, use 2-3 drops in a carrier oil and massage on affected areas. Can also use 3-4 drops in bath water, or use in a hot compress.

To get rid of germs, mix 5-6 drops in a quart of water; pour into a spray bottle. Shake well before using.

To purify air and kill airborne germs, use 2-3 drops in a diffuser.

For detoxification, mix 2-3 drops in a carrier oil, and use in a full body massage. Can also use 3-4 drops in bath water.

To stimulate delayed menstruation, use 2-3 drops in a carrier oil and massage on lower abdomen.

For depression, headaches, mental or nervous exhaustion, and stress, use 2-3 drops in a diffuser, or use 2-3 drops on a handkerchief and periodically inhale.

To relieve menstrual cramps, use 2-3 drops in a carrier oil and massage on lower back and abdomen. Can also be used in a hot compress.

GRAPEFRUIT
(Citrus paradisi)

For acne, place 2-3 drops on a cotton ball and dab affected area. If you have highly sensitive skin, dilute with a carrier oil.

Mixes well with: Basil, cinnamon, clary sage, clove, eucalyptus, frankincense, geranium, ginger, hyssop, jasmine, juniper, lavender, lime, myrrh, neroli, orange, palmarosa, patchouli, peppermint, rosemary, rosewood, sage, sandalwood, tangerine, thyme, and ylang ylang.

Extraction method: Cold expression.

Parts used: Fresh peel.

Safety Information: Has a short shelf-life as it oxidizes quickly. Replace quarterly.

FUN FACT:
In many parts of the world, the waste of grapefruit and other citrus fruits are ground and used as animal feed.

(See Color Photo on Page 73)

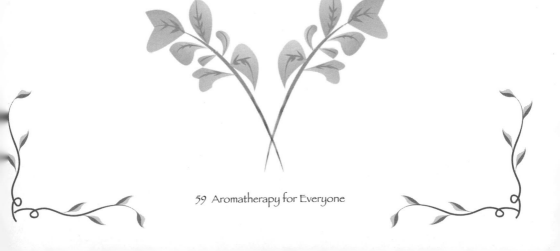

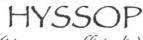

HYSSOP
(Hyssopus officinalis)

Hyssop, also known as the holy herb, is mentioned numerous times in the Holy Bible. Used by powerful biblical leaders, like David, Moses, Solomon, and Jesus, hyssop cleansed and purified mankind, both internally and externally. It was also used to wash and polish sacred places. Others embraced hyssop as well. The Greeks used hyssop for respiratory problems. Persians used hyssop in a type of body lotion to give the skin a fine color. Indians used it to reduce body tissue fluids, to alleviate bruises, and to soothe cuts and wounds. And Europeans in the 17th century used hyssop as an air freshener. Once used extensively across the globe, its use in the Western world diminished as modern day medicine took its place. Now with a resurgence in acceptance of holistic therapies, hyssop is once again a therapeutic leader.

Therapeutic uses: Antiseptic, appetite loss, asthma, anxiety, bloating, bronchitis, bruises, circulation, clarity, concentration, colds and flu, coughs, cuts, creativity, digestive system, eczema, emotional balance, excess phlegm, inflammation (skin), low blood pressure, meditation, menstrual problems, mental fatigue, nervous tension, sore throat, stress-related conditions, tonsillitis, whooping cough, wounds.

Essential Oil Applications:

As an antiseptic, use 2-3 drops on a cotton ball or swab and apply to wounds.

To help relieve anxiety, mental fatigue, nervous tension, and stress-related disorders, and to aid clarity, concentration, and creativity, and for meditation, use 2-3 drops in a diffuser.

For appetite loss, bloating, and poor digestion, add 2-3 drops in a carrier oil and massage over entire abdominal area.

For bronchitis, coughs, excess phlegm, and other respiratory problems, there are three different ways to use hyssop: use 2-3 drops in a diffuser, or combine 2-3 drops in 1 ounce of carrier oil, and rub mixture on chest. Can also place 2-3 drops on a cotton ball or handkerchief and breathe in periodically.

To boost circulation, use 4-6 drops in 2 ounces of carrier oil and massage over entire body.

HYSSOP
(Hyssopus officinalis)

To help heal cuts and wounds, dilute with water, place on cotton ball, and dab affected areas.

If emotions are running wild, use 2-3 drops in a diffuser.

To help with low blood pressure, use 3-5 drops in a diffuser regularly.

For menstrual problems, like bloating and water retention, use 2-3 drops in 1 ounce of carrier oil and massage on lower abdomen and lower back area. Can also use 8-10 drops in bath water.

For sore throats, tonsillitis, or whooping cough, use 3-5 drops in a steam inhalation.

Mixes well with: Clary sage, geranium, grapefruit, lavender, lemon, lime, orange, sage, rosemary, and tangerine.

Extraction method: Steam distillation.

Parts used: Leaves and flowering tops.

Safety Information: Avoid if pregnant. Do not use if diagnosed with epilepsy or high blood pressure.

> ## FUN FACT:
> In the 10th century, Benedictine monks introduced hyssop to Europe as an ingredient for liqueurs.

(See Color Photo on Page 73)

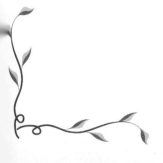

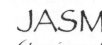

JASMINE
(Jasminum officinale)

Exotic and sweet, jasmine is a highly sought after oil. Exorbitantly expensive in its pure form, it's not uncommon to find "cut" or synthetic versions on the market. These variants are beneficial as well as affordable. Jasmine's historic use goes back centuries. In ancient India, jasmine was (and still is) used for for ceremonial purposes. The Chinese used jasmine to cleanse the atmosphere that surrounded the sick. A good hostess also made sure to have jasmine on hand to give to inebriated guests to clear their heads. Modern uses for jasmine include childbirth, depression, respiration, and fertility.

Therapeutic uses: Confidence, coughs, depression, energy, fertility, labor, libido, menstrual pain, muscle spasm and sprains, nervousness, optimism, postnatal depression, lactation, respiration problems, skin care, tension, vitality, voice loss.

Essential Oil Applications:

To restore confidence, energy, optimism, and vitality, use 3-5 drops in a diffuser. Can also add 8-10 drops to bath water.

For coughs, especially the lingering kind, use 3-5 drops in a steam inhalation.

To alleviate depression, nervousness, and tension, use 3-5 drops in a diffuser. Can also add 8-10 drops to bath water.

To promote male fertility, use regularly in massage (3-5 drops mixed with 1 ounce of carrier oil). Can also add 8-10 drops to bath water or use 3-5 drops in a diffuser.

A bath made with 8-10 drops of oil will help relieve headache, premenstrual syndrome, stress, and tension.

To help strengthen contractions during childbirth and relieve labor pain, use 3-5 drops in a diffuser placed in birthing room. Do not start diffusing oil until labor is well-advanced.

When lactating, jasmine will help promote the flow of breast milk. Use 8-10 drops in bath water, or 3-5 drops in a blended massage oil regularly. Can also use 3-5 drops in a diffuser.

JASMINE
(Jasminum grandiflorum)

To promote libido in both men and women, use 3-5 drops in a diffuser, or 8-10 drops in bath water.

For muscle spasms and sprains, mix 3-5 drops with 1 ounce of carrier oil, and massage on affected areas.

For postnatal depression, mix 3-5 drops in 1 ounce of carrier oil and massage on body. Can also add 8-10 drops to bath water, or use 3-5 drops in a diffuser.

To use as a skin tonic for all skin types, mix a few drops with an application of unscented face lotion. Can also mix with lavender, tangerine, and a carrier oil for a blend that can encourage cell growth and increase elasticity.

To help relieve stress and tension, use 2-3 drops in a diffuser or lamp ring. Can also use 20 drops in 1 ounce of carrier oil for a relaxing massage.

For respiratory problems, use 5 drops in a steam inhalation. Especially good for deepening breathing, and calming spasms of the bronchi.

Mixes well with: Bergamot, clary sage, clove, frankincense, geranium, ginger, grapefruit, lemon, lime, neroli, orange, palmarosa, rose, rosewood, sandalwood, tangerine, and ylang ylang.

Extraction method: Solvent extraction of the flowers can produce both a concrete and an absolute. Jasmine essential oil is produced from the absolute via steam distillation.

Parts used: Flowers.

Safety Information: Avoid during most of pregnancy; do not use until labor is well advanced.

> ## FUN FACT:
> Flowers must be picked before sunrise, and experienced pickers can pick between 10,000 and 15,000 per day.

(See Color Photo on Page 73)

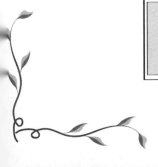

JUNIPER BERRY
(Juniperus communis)

Juniper berry was one of the first aromatics used in ancient civilization, and has a colorful history of use. The ancient Greeks burned juniper branches to combat epidemics. The English burned it as well, and hoped its magical powers would repel evil spirits, witches, and demons. Ancient Egyptians anointed corpses with juniper oil, and used the berries in cosmetics and perfumes. Europeans regarded juniper oil as a miracle cure for typhoid, cholera, dysentery, and tapeworms. Many cultures today still value juniper's many benefits. Tibetans still revere juniper and use it as a purification incense, while Native Americans burn it in their cleansing ceremonies. Holistic medicine also embraces juniper, and considers it a highly versatile and therapeutic oil.

Therapeutic uses: Acne, arthritis, appetite regulator, anxiety, cellulite, colds and flu, detoxify, disinfectant, drowsiness, eczema, gout, hair loss, headaches, immune system, infections, mental exhaustion, menstrual problems, nervous tension, oily complexions, rheumatism, skin toner, stress-related conditions, wounds.

Essential Oil Applications:

For acne, eczema, oily complexions, and wounds, place enough oil on a cotton ball to make it wet, but do not soak it. Wipe directly on skin condition, using gentle movements.

To alleviate anxiety, drowsiness, mental exhaustion, nervous tension, and combat stress-related disorders, use 8-10 drops in bath water. Can also use 2-3 drops in a diffuser.

For arthritis and rheumatism, add 2-3 drops to 1 ounce of carrier oil and massage into affected areas.

As an appetite regulator, use 2-3 drops in a diffuser or use as a steam inhalation.

For cellulite and detoxification, add 2-3 drops to 1 ounce of carrier oil and massage into affected areas regularly. Can also use 8-10 drops in bath water.

JUNIPER BERRY
(Juniperus communis)

To fight colds, flu, and infections, use 3-5 drops in a steam inhalation. Can also use 8-10 drops in bath water, or 3-5 in a diffuser.

To help prevent hair loss, mix 3-5 drops in unscented conditioner. Leave on hair for 3-5 minutes, rinse as normal. Use regularly.

For headaches, use 2-3 drops in a diffuser or 8-10 drops in a bath. Can also use 2-3 drops in one ounce of carrier oil, and massage gently into temples. Increase benefit by adding lavender.

As a home disinfectant, use approx. 5 drops in a quart of water. Transfer to a spray bottle, and shake before using.

To boost the immune system, use 8-10 drops in bath water, or use 2-3 drops in a diffuser.

To regulate period and to fight cramps, use 2-3 drops in one ounce of carrier oil and massage on lower abdomen.

Mixes well with: Atlas cedarwood, bergamot, cedarwood, clary sage, eucalyptus, geranium, ginger, grapefruit, lavender, lime, myrrh, orange, palmarosa, peppermint, pine, rosemary, sandalwood, tangerine, and tea tree.

Extraction method: Steam distillation.

Parts used: Dried, crushed, or slightly dried ripe fruit.

Safety Information: Avoid if pregnant. Do not use if diagnosed with kidney problems.

FUN FACT:
Juniper was once considered to have the power to restore lost youth.

(See Color Photo on Page 73)

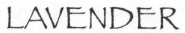

LAVENDER
(Lavandula augustifolia)

Lavender is the most loved aromatic used in aromatherapy today. Besides being versatile, its lightly floral and soothing scent is one that most people find appealing. In therapeutic terms, lavender is the most useful oil, and one that every aromatherapy kit should include. It's also one of the few essential oils that can be applied neat. (Essential oils are highly concentrated plant oils. Read and follow instructions for use carefully.) Lavender has a long history of use in many different cultures, but is probably most associated with the English for its use in many of their perfumes.

Also worthy of mention is the essential oil lavandin *(Lavandula hydrida)*, a hybrid form of lavender. While it provides most of the same benefits as lavender, it is more penetrating and has a sharper scent. These qualities make it perfect to combat respiratory, muscular, and and circulatory ailments.

Therapeutic uses: Acne, alopecia, anxiety, asthma, bee and wasp stings, bronchial problems, depression, eczema, dermatitis, flu symptoms, insect repellent, insomnia, hay fever, headaches, menstruation regulation, migraine, minor cuts and burns, mood swings, nervous tension, nightmares, psoriasis, rashes, sleep aid, stress, sunburn.

Essential Oil Applications:

For skin problems, including acne, dermatitis, eczema, psoriasis, rashes, and sunburn, place 2-3 drops on a cotton ball and dab on affected area.

As a tonic for hair growth, mix 2-3 drops in a quarter-sized application of unscented, leave-on conditioner and massage into scalp.

To alleviate headaches and migraines, massage a couple of drops into temples. Can also use in a hot or cold compress.

To relieve insomnia or aid sleep, use 2-3 drops in a diffuser, or place same amount on a cotton ball or handkerchief, and place inside pillowcase. Can also use 8-10 drops in a bath before bedtime.

For anxiety, depression, nervous tension, stress, or to balance mood

LAVENDER
(Lavandula officinalis)

swings, use 2-3 drops in a diffuser. Can also use 8-10 drops in a bath. To guard against nightmares, use 8-10 drops in a bath before bedtime.

For menstrual regulation or PMS, use 4-5 drops in 1 ounce of carrier oil and massage on abdomen and lower back.

For bee and wasp stings, place 2-3 drops on a cotton ball and dab on affected area.

To lessen flu symptoms, use 2-3 drops in a diffuser, or as a steam inhalation.

To repel moths, use several drops on cotton balls, and place strategically in linen closet and/or wardrobe.

For asthma, bronchial problems, and hay fever, use 2-3 drops in a diffuser or as a steam inhalation. Can also use 8-10 drops in bath, or use 4-5 drops in 1 ounce of carrier oil and rub on chest area.

Mixes well with: Almost all oils, and particularly well with allspice, anise, basil, bergamot, citronella, chamomile, clary sage, clove, eucalyptus, frankincense, geranium, grapefruit, hyssop, jasmine, juniper, lemon, lime, tangerine, patchouli, peppermint, pine, rose, rosemary, spearmint, tea tree, and thyme.

Extraction method: Steam distillation

Parts used: Fresh flowering tops.

Safety Information: Can make those with low blood pressure drowsy.

FUN FACT:
In the 12th century, German herbalist Hildegarde von Bingen declared that lavender was good for maintaining a pure character.

(See Color Photo on Page 74)

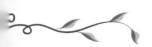

LEMON
(Citrus limon)

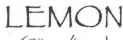

have long been valued for more than lemonade. We know cient Egyptians prized this oil for its purported ability to act as an antidote to fish and meat poisoning. And, like lime, it was a staple on 17th century Royal Navy ships to help prevent scurvy. Today, we know lemon can help contain and treat infectious diseases, especially colds and fevers. Its scent also helps to increase concentration, and neutralizes unpleasant odors. Some hospitals use lemon oil to help calm frightened or depressed patients. It also boosts the immune system by stimulating production of white and red blood cells. Lemon oil is a must for every aromatherapy kit.

Therapeutic uses: Air freshener, anemia, circulation, colds and flu, constipation, corns, coughs, dandruff, depression, digestive system, dull complexion, emotional confusion, fatigue, fingernail toughener, greasy hair & skin, hypertension, household cleanser, immune booster, insect repellent, joint pain, low energy, listlessness, mouth ulcers, nosebleed, PMS, scars, stress, throat infections, voice loss, warts.

Essential Oil Applications:

To freshen air and neutralize bad odors, use 2-3 drops in a diffuser. While cleaning, add 2-3 drops to rinse water to wipe away greasy residue and for extra freshness.

For anemia and high blood pressure, use 2-3 drops in a diffuser regularly. Can also use as a steam inhalation.

For joint pain, use 2-3 drops in 1 ounce of carrier oil and massage on affected area. Can also add 8-10 drops in bath water.

For circulatory health, mix 2-3 drops in 1 ounce of carrier oil and massage on body. Can also use 8-10 drops in bath water, or a few drops in a steam inhalation.

For colds, coughs, flu, and voice loss, use 2-3 drops in a steam inhalation. Also add to carrier oil and rub on chest and neck. To cool fever, use 2-3 drops in a cold compress. After an illness, use 2-3 drops in a diffuser or steam inhalation as a tonic for the immune system. Continue use for 2-3 days.

LEMON
(Citrus limon)

For corns and warts, use neat on a cotton swab and apply directly to affected area. Be careful not to apply to surrounding area.

To alleviate emotional distress, confusion, fatigue, PMS, and stress, use 2-3 drops in a diffuser. Can use 8-10 drops in bath water.

To boost digestive health, use 2-3 drops regularly in steam inhaler or diffuser.

To toughen fingernails, mix 2-3 drops in 1 ounce of almond oil and massage into cuticles and on fingernails regularly.

For mouth ulcers or throat infections, use in mouthwash. Swish, gargle, and rinse with water. Use regularly until condition has abated.

For nosebleeds, place a few drops on a cotton ball and inhale.

For greasy hair, mix 2-3 drops with unscented shampoo. For greasy skin, mix 2-3 drops of oil in 1 oz. of water. Mix well, place on cotton ball. Apply to skin as a toner.

As insect repellent, use 2-3 drops in diffuser or add a few drops to cotton ball, and place in infested areas.

To soften scar tissue, mix 2-3 drops in 1 oz. of carrier oil. Massage on scar regularly.

Does Not Mix well with: allspice, anise seed, atlas cedar, camphor, chamomile, clove, lime, nutmeg, patchouli, pennyroyal, spearmint, wintergreen.

Extraction method: Cold expression.

Parts used: Outer part of fresh peel.

Safety Information: May cause skin irritation in sensitive people. Avoid direct sunlight after use, as it may have a mild phototoxic effect.

> **FUN FACT:** In Japan, lemon essential oil is used throughout banks everywhere, in order to reduce worker error.

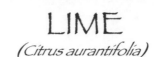

LIME
(Citrus aurantifolia)

Fruity and refreshing, limes have been a kitchen staple for centuries. It is believed that limes were first introduced to the Americas by 16th century Portuguese navigators. The lime soon became a favorite fruit, both for its therapeutic value and taste. Traditionally, lime has been used as a remedy for indigestion, heartburn, and nausea. It also has cooling effects on fevers, and can help ease coughs and various respiratory disorders. Lime oil is also useful as part of a beauty regimen, as its astringic properties help clear oily skin and acne. Plus, because lime oil also promotes good circulation, it is often used to help relieve varicose veins. Last but not least, lime oil has a wonderfully uplifting scent, with the power to uplift and re-energize the spirit.

Therapeutic uses: Acne, arthritis, cellulite, chest congestion, colds, coughs, cuts, deodorant, depression, disinfectant, exhaustion, fevers, general cleaning, immune system tonic, listlessness, nail growth, rheumatism, sinusitis, sore throats, varicose veins, wounds.

Essential Oil Applications:

For acne, mix 2-3 drops of oil in 1 ounce of water. Mix well, then place on cotton ball. Gently apply to affected area. Can also be used as a toner for oily skin.

For arthritis and rheumatism, use 2-3 drops in 1 ounce of carrier oil and massage on affected area.

For bleeding cuts and wounds, use 2-3 drops of oil in a cold compress.

For cellulite, mix 2-3 drops in 1 ounce of carrier oil, and massage on affected area regularly.

For chest congestion, colds, coughs, sinusitis, and sore throats, use 2-3 drops in a steam inhalation. Can also be added to a carrier oil and rubbed on chest and neck.

To alleviate depression, exhaustion, and listlessness, use 2-3 drops in a diffuser. Can use 8-10 drops in bath water.

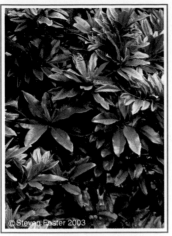

Allspice

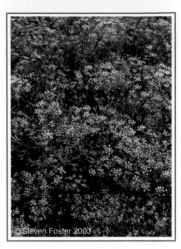

Anise

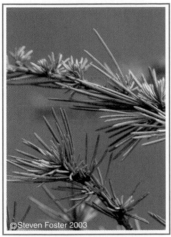

Atlas Cedar

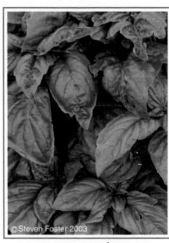

Basil

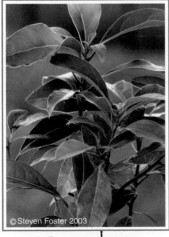

Camphor

71

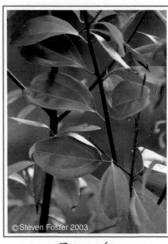

Cassia

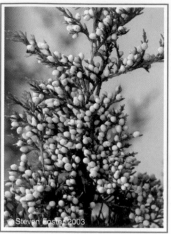

Cedarwood

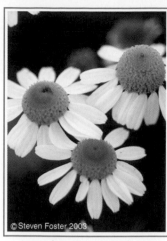

Chamomile

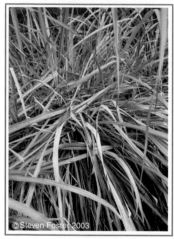

Citronella

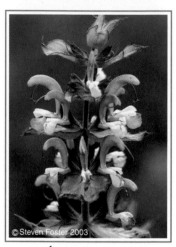

Clary Sage

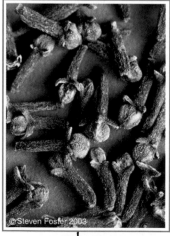

Clove

72

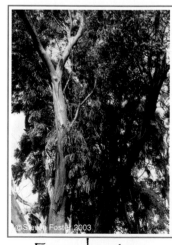

Eucalyptus

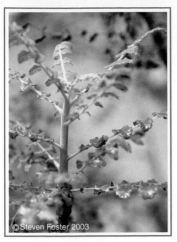

Frankinsence

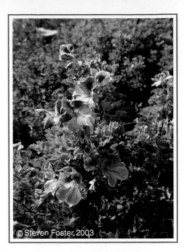

Geranium

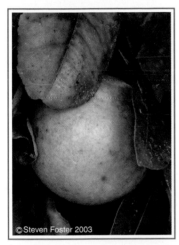

Grapefruit

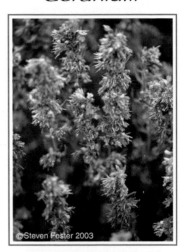

Hyssop

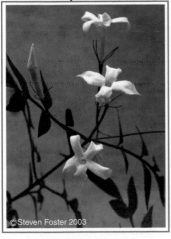

Jasmine

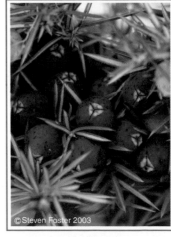

Juniper

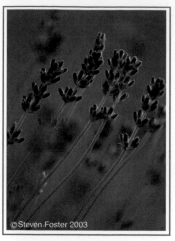

Lavender

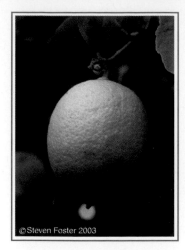

Lemon

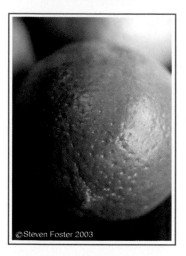

Lime

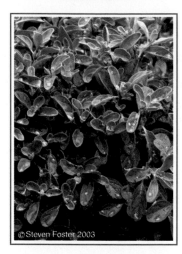

Marjoram

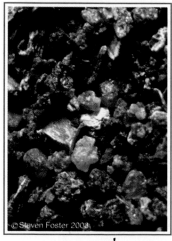

Myrrh

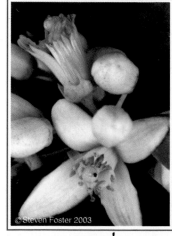

Neroli

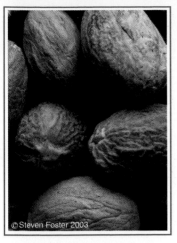

Nutmeg

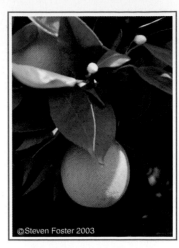

Orange

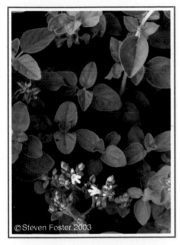

Oregano

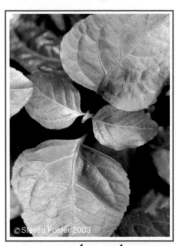

Patchouli

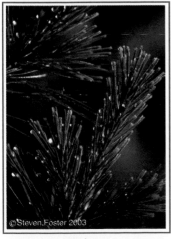

Pine

75

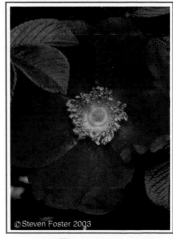

Rose

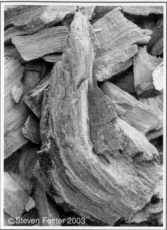

Sandalwood

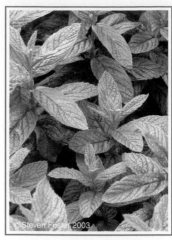

Spearmint

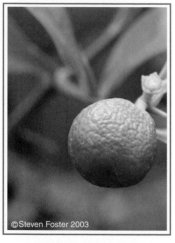

Tangerine

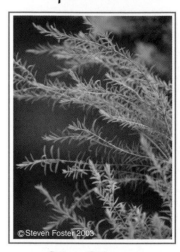

Tea Tree

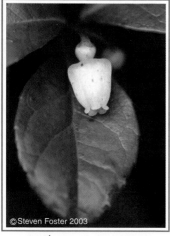

Wintergreen

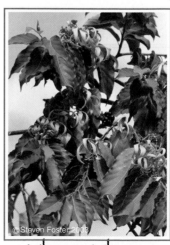

Ylang-Ylang

LIME
(Citrus aurantifolia)

As a deodorant, mix 2-3 drops in 1 ounce of water. Dab on with a cotton ball. For extra deodorant protection in bath, put unscented shower gel in palm of hand, mix in a drop or two of oil, and shower as normal.

As a disinfectant, add 5-6 drops in a quart-sized spray bottle of water. Shake well before using. Refresh weekly.

To cool fever, use 2-3 drops in a cold compress.

After an illness, use 2-3 drops in a diffuser or steam inhalation as a tonic for the immune system. Continue use for 2-3 days.

To promote nail growth, mix 2-3 drops in 1 ounce of almond oil and massage into cuticles.

While cleaning refrigerator, freezer, or oven, add 2-3 drops to rinse water to wipe away greasy residue and for extra freshness.

For varicose veins, mix 2-3 drops in a carrier oil and massage on affected area.

Mixes well with: Basil, bergamot, citronella, clary sage, eucalyptus, geranium, ginger, grapefruit, hyssop, jasmine, juniper, lavender, neroli, nutmeg, rosemary, rosewood, sage, sandalwood, tangerine, and ylang ylang.

Extraction method: Cold expression or steam distillation.

Parts used: Peel of unripe fruit (cold expression), whole ripe crushed fruit (steam distillation).

Safety Information: May cause photosensitivity in strong sunlight; use in moderation.

FUN FACT:
In the 17th century, English sailors ate limes to prevent scurvy, a disease caused by a deficiency of vitamin C. Soon afterward, the English were dubbed "limeys," a colorful nickname which has survived throughout all these years.

(See Color Photo on Page 74)

MARJORAM
(Origanum majorana)

Its fresh, warm, and slightly woody aroma reflects the meaning of marjoram's botanical name: joy of the mountain. This popular herb has been used therapeutically for centuries. Ancient Greeks used it to calm muscle spasms, relieve excess fluid in the tissues, and also as an antidote to poison. Greek women also used an oil made with marjoram on their heads as a relaxant. In 16th century Europe, the herb was scattered on the floors of rooms everywhere to mask unpleasant smells. Today, while marjoram may be best known for lending a unique flavor to foods, it's also a favorite of aromatherapists everywhere. With therapeutic value to win challenges from ailments like anxiety and high blood pressure, marjoram is a valuable and pleasing aromatic to have on hand.

Therapeutic uses: Anxiety, arthritis, asthma, bronchitis, bruises, chillblains, colds, coughs, digestive problems (flatulence, constipation, indigestion), grief, headaches, high blood pressure, hyperactivity, insomnia, lumbago, menstrual cramps, migraines, muscular aches and stiffness, premenstrual syndrome, nervous tension, rheumatism, seasickness, sprains, stress.

Essential Oil Applications:

For anxiety, grief, hyperactivity, insomnia, nervous tension, and stress, use 2-3 drops in a diffuser, or add 8-10 drops in bath water before bedtime.

For arthritis, lumbago, muscular aches and stiffness, rheumatism, and sprains, use 2-3 drops in 1 ounce of carrier oil and massage affected areas. Can also be used in a hot or cold compress as needed.

For asthma, bronchitis, colds, and coughs, use 2-3 drops in 1 ounce of carrier oil and rub on chest and throat. Can also use 2-3 drops in a steam inhalation.

For bruises or chillblains, use 2-3 drops in a carrier oil and dab on area. Can also be used neat, but just on affected area. (Essential oils are highly concentrated plant oils. Read and follow instructions for use carefully.)

For digestive problems, like constipation, indigestion, and flatulence, use 2-3 drops in a carrier oil and massage on back.

MARJORAM
(Thymus mastichina)

For high blood pressure, use 2-3 drops in a carrier oil and use in a full-body massage. Can also use 8-10 drops in a bath.

For headaches and migraines, use 2-3 drops in a carrier oil and massage on temples and neck. Can also be used in a hot or cold compress.

For menstrual cramps and premenstrual syndrome, use 2-3 drops in a carrier oil and massage on lower abdomen and lower back. Can also be used as a hot compress, or use 8-10 drops in bath water.

For seasickness, use 2-3 drops on a handkerchief; inhale periodically.

Mixes well with: Atlas cedarwood, bergamot, cinnamon, clary sage, eucalyptus, lavender, lemon, orange, pine, tangerine, rosemary, rosewood, tea tree, thyme, and ylang ylang.

Extraction method: Steam distillation.

Parts used: Fresh and dried leaves and flowering tops.

Safety Information: Avoid if pregnant. Not suitable for small children. If diagnosed with depression, do not use as it has a strong, sedative effect. Excessive use may cause drowsiness.

FUN FACT:
To suppress sexual desire and impulses, many religious institutions used marjoram for its anti-aphrodisiac affect.

(See Color Photo on Page 74)

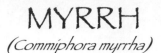

MYRRH
(Commiphora myrrha)

Best known for its presentation as a gift to the baby Jesus, myrrh appeared several more times in the Holy Bible. Myrhh has been in use for its therapeutic value for over 3,000 years, and continues to be a powerhouse in the world of holistic medicine. Ancient Egyptians used myrrh to treat herpes and hay fever. Myrrh was also important to Greek soldiers who took myrrh into the battlefield with them, as its antiseptic and anti-inflammatory properties made it helpful for cleaning and healing wounds. Even today, healers all over the world are still using it. Tibetans use myrrh to help alleviate stress and nervous disorders, while the Chinese use it for arthritis, menstrual problems, sores, and hemorrhoids. Warm, rich, and spicy in scent, myrrh is a welcome addition to every aromatherapy kit.

Therapeutic uses: Appetite, anger, asthma, athlete's foot, bedsores, boils, bronchitis, chapped skin, colds, coughs, digestive system, eczema, gingivitis, hemorrhoids, mouth ulcers, rejuvenate mature complexions, rheumatism, skin ulcers, sore throats, sores, spongy gums, stress, viral infections, wounds, wrinkles.

Essential Oil Applications:

To restore appetite and calm the digestive system, use 2-3 drops in a diffuser or steam inhalation. Can also be added to a carrier oil and massaged on abdomen.

To calm anger and stress, use 2-3 drops in a diffuser.

For asthma, coughs, colds, and sore throats, use 2-3 drops in 1 ounce of carrier oil. Rub on chest for asthma, coughs, and cold, and on throat if sore. Can also use 2-3 drops in a diffuser or steam inhalation.

For athlete's foot, bedsores, boils, skin ulcers, sores, and wounds, use 2-3 drops in a cold compress and apply to affected area. Can also be added to a cotton ball and dabbed on directly; use lightly.

For chapped skin or hemorrhoids, add 2-3 drops to 2 tablespoons of liquid lanolin, and massage into affected areas.

For mouth disorders, like gingivitis, mouth ulcers, and spongy gums, mix 2-3 drops in a glass of water and swish in mouth. Spit out.

MYRRH
(Commiphora myrrha)

To rejuvenate mature complexions and to smooth out wrinkles, wash face, then use 2-3 drops with 1 ounce of almond carrier oil, and rub gently onto face.

Mixes well with: Allspice, basil, bergamot, clove, frankincense, geranium, ginger, grapefruit, juniper, lavender, lemon, nutmeg, palmarosa, patchouli, peppermint, pine, rosemary, sandalwood, spearmint, tangerine, tea tree, thyme, and ylang ylang.

Extraction method: Steam distillation.

Parts used: Oleoresin-gum

Safety Information: Avoid if pregnant. Do not use in high concentrations.

FUN FACT:
According to Greek mythology, Aphrodite transformed Myrrha, the daughter of the king of Cypress, into a shrub (Commiphora myrrha) as punishment for sexual deviancy.

(See Color Photo on Page 74)

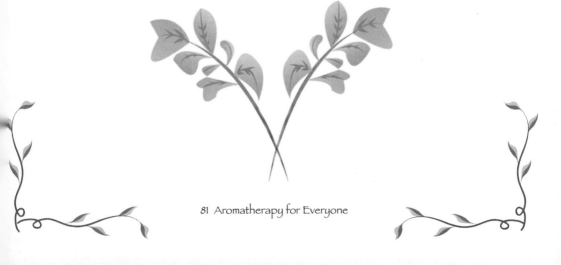

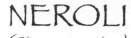

NEROLI
(Citrus aurantium)

Neroli oil is heady, sweet, and floral, and is made from the aromatic blossoms of the orange tree. It's rare to find a pure 100% neroli oil, as it's impossible for companies to be able to offer it for a low cost. It takes approximately 1,000 pounds of orange blossoms to make one pound of neroli oil. Therefore, it is not unusual to find it "cut" with another oil. This is perfectly acceptable, and does not reduce neroli's benefits at all. Used for centuries to combat plague, fever, and nervousness, neroli is a one of the most user-friendly oils there is. It helps regenerate skin cells, improves skin elasticity, and even helps with acne, scarring, and stretch marks. Internally, neroli acts as a natural tranquilizer, and can relieve chronic anxiety, depression, and stress. Besides being a beloved oil by aromatherapists all over the globe, neroli is also often used in bridal bouquets, both as a symbol of purity, and for its ability to calm the bride's nerves.

Therapeutic uses: Acne, antispasmodic, anxiety, aphrodisiac, circulation, depression, headaches, hysteria, insomnia, lethargy, mature skin, menopause, neuralgia, panic, premenstrual discomfort, scars, shock, stress, stretch marks.

Essential Oil Applications:

For acne, wet a cotton ball, then apply a few drops of oil. Dab affected area lightly.

To fight lethargy, use 2-3 drops in a diffuser.

As an antispasmodic, use 2-3 drops in a diffuser or 4-5 drops in a blended massage to improve colon problems, diarrhea, and nervous dyspepsia.

To alleviate anxiety, depression, hysteria, lethargy, panic, shock, and stress, use 3-4 drops in a diffuser. Can also use 8-10 drops in bath water.

To improve circulation, mix 3-4 drops in 1 ounce of carrier oil and massage on body. Can also use 8-10 drops in bath water regularly.

For headaches and neuralgia, use 3-4 drops in a hot or cold compress (whichever works best for you).

NEROLI
(Citrus aurantium)

To ease premenstrual discomfort and distress, use 3-4 drops in a diffuser or 8-10 drops in bath water.

To regenerate skin cells and improve skin elasticity for mature skin, mix a drop or two with an application of an unscented face cream, and apply as normal.

To help with the irritability and tearfulness that can accompany menopause, use 3-4 drops in a diffuser or 8-10 drops in bath water regularly. Can also mix 3-4 drops with 1 ounce of carrier oil and massage on body.

To help diminish scars and stretch marks, mix 3-4 drops with liquid lanolin and massage into affected areas.

Mixes well with: Bergamot, frankincense, geranium, grapefruit, jasmine, lavender, lemon, lime, orange, rose, rosemary, sandalwood, tangerine, and ylang ylang.

Extraction method: Steam distillation or enfleurage.

Part used: Orange blossom petals.

Safety Information: Because of its calming and almost tranquilizing affect, do not use when a clear head is needed, or before driving a vehicle or operating other heavy machinery.

FUN FACT:
It is believed that neroli was named after Princess Anne Marie of Nerola, who loved to wear this sweet, floral scented oil as a perfume.

(See Color Photo on Page 74)

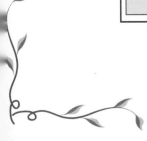

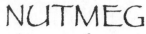

NUTMEG
(Myristica fragrans)

Nutmeg is valued by great cooks everywhere for its versatility in the kitchen. It's nutty, spicy, and slightly sweet taste makes it a valuable ingredient in everything from meat dishes to desserts. So prized was nutmeg that in the Middle Ages the Dutch plotted extreme measures to keep the price high, while the English and French hatched their own counterplots to obtain fertile seeds so they could cultivate it themselves.

Besides its culinary uses, nutmeg is also a highly valued aromatic. The Romans used it as incense, and the Egyptians for embalming. Indians found nutmeg to be perfect for intestinal disorders, and Italians found it useful in combating the Plague. In the Middle Ages, nutmeg was grated and used with lard as an ointment for hemorrhoids. Today, nutmeg is used in aromatherapy for a variety of ailments, from circulatory problems to boosting libido.

Therapeutic uses: Appetite, arthritis, bad breath, circulation, digestive problems, fainting spell, gout, impotence, libido, muscle pain, nervous fatigue, rheumatism.

Essential Oil Applications:

For arthritis, gout, muscle pain, and rheumatism, use 2-3 drops in a carrier oil and massage on affected area. Can also be used in a diffuser.

To stimulate appetite, use 2-3 drops in a diffuser.

For bad breath, use a few drops in water as a mouthwash.

For circulatory health, mix 2-3 drops in a carrier oil and massage all over body.

For digestive problems, use 8-10 drops in bath water. Can also use 2-3 drops in a diffuser.

To revive after a fainting spell, use 2-3 drops on a cotton ball or handkerchief; place under nose of the person who fainted.

NUTMEG
(Myristica fragrans)

For hemorrhoids, mix 2-3 drops of oil with 2 tablespoons of liquid lanolin. Apply to affected area. Can also add to a carrier oil.

For nervous fatigue, use 2-3 drops in a diffuser, or add 8-10 drops in bath water.

For impotence and to revive libido, use 6-8 drops in a bath.

Mixes well with: Bergamot, clary sage, clove, geranium, lime, myrrh, orange, rosemary, tangerine, and tea tree.

Extraction method: Steam or water distillation.

Parts used: Dried worm-eaten nutmeg seed (worms eat all the starch and fat content).

Safety Information: Avoid if pregnant. Very large doses can cause nausea or stupor.

FUN FACT:
Yankee peddlers used to sell unsuspecting housewives fake "nutmegs" whittled from wood, bilking them out of money and leaving town before being found out.

(See Color Photo on Page 75)

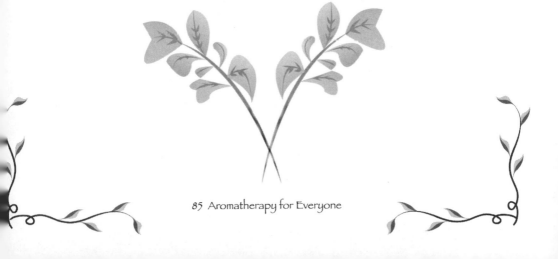

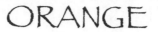

ORANGE

(Citrus sinensis)

Orange oil is one of the best aromatics for the beginner. Besides lending a quality ambiance to any environment, orange oil is basically foolproof to use. It mixes well with many essential oils, plus softens and warms up the blend. It also has a variety of therapeutic uses, from relaxing mind and spirit to boosting circulation to protecting wood. It's user-friendly in nature, and inexpensive to keep on hand. Historically, oranges have been associated with generosity and gratitude, and symbolized innocence and fertility. Native to China and India, oranges are now grown in abundance in the Americas, Israel, and the Mediterranean.

Therapeutic uses: Acne, blemishes, boredom, bronchitis, cellulite, chills, chronic fatigue syndrome, colds, constipation, coughs, creativity, depression, disinfectant, eczema, fear, fever, flu, fluid retention, gingivitis, joint pain, lethargy, mental exhaustion, mouth ulcers, muscle pain, nervous anxiety, oily skin, premenstrual syndrome, psoriasis, seasonal affective disorder, skin care, stress.

Essential Oil Applications:

For acne, blemishes, and to combat oily skin, wet a cotton ball and add 2 drops oil. Dab lightly on acne and blemishes, or gently rub off facial oils.

To fight against boredom and lethargy, use 2-3 drops in a diffuser.

For cellulite, mix 2-3 drops with 1 ounce of carrier oil and massage into affected area regularly.

To cool a fever or warm a chill, use in a compress: cold for a fever, hot for a chill. Can also use 8-10 drops in bath water, or add 2-3 drops in 1 ounce of carrier oil and use in a massage.

For colds, coughs, and flu, use 2-3 drops in a steam inhalation. Can also use 2-3 drops in a carrier oil and rub on chest.

For constipation, add 2-3 drops to 1 ounce of carrier oil and massage into lower back area.

To inspire creativity, use 2-3 drops in a diffuser.

ORANGE
(Citrus sinensis)

For chronic fatigue syndrome, depression, fear, mental exhaustion, nervous tension, and stress, use 2-3 drops in a diffuser or steam inhalation. Can also use 8-10 drops in bath water.

To alleviate fluid retention, use 2-3 drops in a carrier oil and massage on lower abdomen and back. Can also be massaged on other affected areas.

For gingivitis and mouth ulcers, place 2-3 drops in a glass, add water and mix. Swish around mouth, spit out. Repeat as necessary.

For joint and muscle pain, use 2-3 drops in a carrier oil and massage on affected area. Can also be used in a hot compress.

To reduce inflammation associated with eczema and psoriasis, use 2-3 drops in a carrier oil and massage on affected area.

To help alleviate stress brought on by seasonal affective disorder and premenstrual syndrome, use 2-3 drops in a diffuser. Can also use 8-10 drops in bath water.

Mixes well with: Almost all essential oils, but especially well with allspice, anise, basil, bergamot, cinnamon, citronella, clary sage, clove, eucalyptus, frankincense, geranium, ginger, grapefruit, hyssop, jasmine, juniper, lemon, marjoram, oregano, neroli, nutmeg, palmarosa, patchouli, rosewood, sage, sandalwood, and ylang ylang.

Extraction method: Cold-pressed.

Part used: Orange peel.

Safety Information: Do not apply before going out into sunlight. Highly sensitive people should perform a patch test.

> ### FUN FACT:
> On Chinese New Year, oranges are given as gifts to symbolize happiness and prosperity.

(See Color Photo on Page 75)

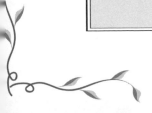

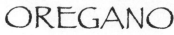

OREGANO
(Origanum vulgare)

Probably best known as a workaholic in the kitchen, oregano also has many valuable therapeutic uses. In fact, it may well have first been used for its curative properties before its seasoning properties were discovered. Ancient Egyptians prized oregano for its ability to disinfect wounds and speed up the healing process. It's also believed that they used it in mummification. Throughout the centuries, oregano has been used to sooth coughs, calm digestive disorders, relax tension, and relieve insomnia. As far as kitchen use, it was the Roman gourmet Apicius who loudly proclaimed oregano to be an important part of his culinary creations, leading it to play an important part in Mediterranean cuisine. When GIs returned from overseas after World War II, they demanded to have Mediterranean herb staple in their dishes back home. Their insistence on enjoying this herb is what helped to make it popular in the United States. Today, oregano not only reigns in the kitchen, but also rules in the world of aromatherapy.

Therapeutic uses: Allergies, antiseptic, antiviral, appetite, arthritis, asthma, backache, bronchitis, carpal tunnel syndrome, chronic fatigue syndrome, cellulite, colds, congestion, flu, fungal infections, headaches, immune booster, indigestion, insomnia, lymphatic circulation, menstruation, menstrual cramps, migraines, muscular pain, nervous tension, rheumatism, sprains, swelling.

Essential Oil Applications:

For allergies, asthma, bronchitis, and congestion, use 2-3 drops in 1 ounce of carrier oil and rub on chest and throat. Can also use 2-3 drops in a steam inhalation.

For arthritis, backache, carpal tunnel syndrome, muscular pain, and rheumatism, use 2-3 drops in a carrier oil and massage on affected area.

For chronic fatigue syndrome, insomnia, and nervous tension, use 2-3 drops in a diffuser, or add 8-10 drops in bath water before bedtime.

For cellulite, use 2-3 drops in 1 ounce of carrier oil and massage on affected area regularly.

OREGANO
(Origanum vulgare)

For fungal infections, mix 2-3 drops in 1 ounce of carrier oil, and massage into affected area. Repeat as needed.

For headaches and migraines, use 2-3 drops in a carrier oil and massage on temples and neck. Can also be used in a hot or cold compress.

For indigestion, use 2-3 drops in 1 ounce of carrier oil and rub on chest and abdomen.

To encourage menstruation or to alleviate premenstrual syndrome, use 2-3 drops in a carrier oil and massage on lower abdomen and lower back. Can also be used as a hot compress, or use 8-10 drops in bath water.

To boost lymphatic circulation, use 2-3 drops in a carrier oil and massage into body.

For sprains and swelling, use 2-3 drops in a cold compress.

To boost immunity after sickness, use 2-3 drops in a diffuser.

Mixes well with: Atlas cedar, basil, bergamot, citronella, eucalyptus, lavender, lemon, orange, rosemary, tea tree, thyme, and wintergreen.

Extraction method: Steam distillation.

Parts used: Dried, herb and leaves.

Safety Information: Avoid if pregnant.

> ## FUN FACT:
> The Greek philosopher Aristotle noticed that tortoises who ate snakes, then ate oregano. This appeared to prevent them from being poisoned, so he began to recommend it as an antidote for poison.

(See Color Photo on Page 75)

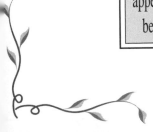

PALMAROSA
(Cymbopogon martinii)

Native to India, palmarosa oil has a rose-like scent, which makes it a popular ingredient in soaps, perfumes, and cosmetics. Palmarosa oil also has a variety of therapeutic uses, and is especially beneficial in skin care because of its moisturizing properties. It stimulates cell regeneration and regulates sebum production, giving it age-defying properties. Additionally, palmarosa oil is great for the digestive system, and was added to Indian curry dishes and West African meat dishes to kill bacteria and aid digestion. Aromatherapists love palmarosa for its skin conditioning properties, and its calming, floral scent.

Therapeutic uses: Acne, colds and flu, cuts, eczema, fatigue, fever, fungal infections (like athlete's foot), intestinal infections, nervousness, physical exhaustion, scars, stress and stress-related conditions, tissue regeneration, wounds.

Essential Oil Applications:

For acne, eczema, and fungal infections, mix 2-3 drops in 1 ounce of carrier oil. Use a cotton ball and swab on affected area. Can also be used neat. (Essential oils are highly concentrated plant oils. Read and follow instructions for use carefully.)

To ease the discomfort of colds and flu, use 2-3 drops in a diffuser.

To accelerate healing of cuts and wounds, place 2-3 drops on a wet cotton ball and dab gently on affected area. This method will also help alleviate scarring.

For fatigue, nervousness, physical exhaustion, stress and stress-related conditions, use 2-3 drops in a diffuser. Can also use 8-10 drops in a bath or 2-3 drops in 1 ounce of carrier oil and massage into body.

To cool a fever, use 2-3 drops in a cold compress. Can also use 8-10 drops in bath.

For intestinal infections, use 3-5 drops in a steam inhalation.

To stimulate sebum production in dry or mature skin, use 2-3 drops in a carrier oil, and dab gently on skin. Can also be used neat. (Essential

PALMAROSA
(Cymbopogon martinii)

oils are highly concentrated plant oils. Read and follow instructions for use carefully.)

Mixes well with: Bergamot, cedarwood, clary sage, clove, geranium, ginger, grapefruit, jasmine, juniper, lavender, lemon, myrrh, orange, patchouli, rose, rosemary, sandalwood, tangerine, thyme, and ylang ylang.

Extraction method: Steam or water distillation.

Parts used: Fresh or dried grass.

Safety Information: No known contraindications, however it's always best to use a patch test before using on skin.

FUN FACT:
Palmarosa oil is used to flavor tobacco.

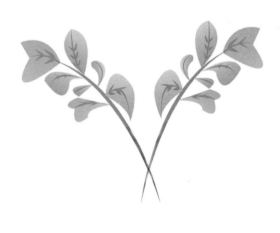

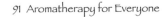

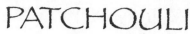

PATCHOULI
(Pogostemon cablin)

Chances are the word "patchouli" brings to mind hippies, free love, and an era of liberation. However, patchouli was used in the East long before the 1970's to scent clothes and linen. In the 19th century, the British learned to identify patchouli as it was used to scent imported fabrics from India. While the musky, earthy scent of patchouli is most associated with fabrics, it has therapeutic properties as well. It's an insect repellent, aphrodisiac, anti-inflammatory, antibacterial, and antifungal. It provides harmony to the body and spirit, and can even fight off body odor by performing as both a deodorant and anti-perspirant. It also has the ability to diminish appetite, making it a friend to dieters all over the globe. Patchouli also has the rare distinction of actually improving with age; the older the oil, the more fuller the scent. Patchouli: it's not just for hippies anymore.

Therapeutic uses: Acne, antiperspirant, anxiety, athlete's foot and other fungal infections, constipation, dandruff, deodorant, dermatitis, eczema, frigidity, insect bites, insect repellent, impotence, libido, loose skin, oily hair and skin, sexual anxiety, stress-related emotional disorders, water retention, weight loss, wounds.

Essential Oil Applications:

For acne, dermatitis, and eczema, mix 2-3 drops with a carrier oil and dab on affected area. Can also be used neat. (Essential oils are highly concentrated plant oils. Read and follow instructions for use carefully.)

As an antiperspirant or deodorant, put 2-3 drops on a cotton ball and dab on underarms.

For athlete's foot and other fungal infections, put 2-3 drops on a cotton ball and dab on affected area.

To alleviate anxiety, add 8-10 drops to bath water. Can also use 2-3 drops in a diffuser.

For dandruff, mix 2-3 drops in unscented conditioner and apply to scalp. Leave on for 3-5 minutes, then rinse.

For constipation, add 8-10 drops in bath water and take a nice, long soak.

To repel insects, use 2-3 drops in a diffuser. Can also be used on a cotton ball, then placed in a linen closet.

PATCHOULI
(Pogostemon patchouli)

For insect bites, use 2-3 drops on a cotton ball; dab on affected area.
To balance libido, fight frigidity and impotence, and to ease sexual anxiety,

To tighten loose skin, especially after weight loss, use 2-3 drops in 1 ounce of carrier oil and massage on body regularly. Can also use 8-10 drops in bath water.

For oily skin, put 2-3 drops on a wet cotton ball and dab on skin. For oily hair, add 2-3 drops to a nickel-sized amount of unscented shampoo. Shampoo as normal; rinse.

To help alleviate stress-related emotional disorders, use 2-3 drops in a diffuser.

To complement a diet and exercise regimen, use 2-3 drops in a diffuser regularly to reduce appetite. Can also use 8-10 drops in a bath.

To ease water retention, use 8-10 drops in bath water or mix 2-3 drops with 1 ounce of carrier oil and massage on body.

To clean wounds, put 2-3 drops on a wet cotton ball and dab affected area gently.

Mixes well with: Allspice, Atlas cedarwood, bergamot, cedarwood, cinnamon, clary sage, frankincense, geranium, ginger, grapefruit, lavender, orange, myrrh, palmarosa, pine, rose, rosewood, sandalwood, tangerine, and ylang ylang.

Extraction method: Steam distillation.

Parts used: Non-flower leaves.

Safety Information: Can be sedative if used in large amounts. Because patchouli can cause appetite loss, do not use if recovering from illness or if battling eating disorders.

FUN FACT:
In Victorian England, people would buy imported Indian cashmere shawls only if they smelled like patchouli. Its scent proved the shawls had been protected from moths during shipment.

(See Color Photo on Page 75)

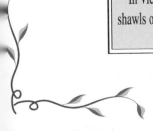

PENNYROYAL
(Mentha pulegium)

Pennyroyal is a member of the mint family, and exudes a fresh, minty, herbaceous scent. While its scent is actually a bit more powerful than other mints, its therapeutic value is actually not as strong. Pennyroyal was used frequently by Ancients for a variety of ailments, and remains current in the British Herbal Pharmacopoeia, which recommends it for flatulence, intestinal colic, the common cold, delayed menstruation, and gout. However, its primary use in today's world of aromatherapy is in pet care. Pennyroyal was a favorite of Pliny the Elder in the fight against fleas, and remains a favorite natural enemy of fleas to this day.

Therapeutic uses: Colds, delayed menstruation, excessive sweating, flatulence, gout, insect repellent, and intestinal colic.

Essential Oil Applications:

For colds, use 2-3 drops in a diffuser.

For delayed menstruation, use 2-3 drops in one ounce of carrier oil and massage on lower abdomen. DO NOT USE if there is any chance of pregnancy.

For excessive sweating, use 2-3 drops in a carrier oil, and dab on underarms.

For flatulence, gout, and intestinal colic, use 2-3 drops in a diffuser.

To protect your dog or cat from fleas, place a few drops on their collar; wait for it to dry before placing around pet's neck. Can also add 2-3 drops to pet shampoo; be sure to rinse pet thoroughly after shampooing.

As an insect repellent, place a few drops of oil on a cotton ball, and place in infested areas. Do not place in areas where a pet could easily find them.

Mixes well with: Citronella, geranium, rosemary, and sage.

Extraction method: Steam distillation.

PENNYROYAL
(Mentha pulegium)

Parts used: Fresh or slightly dried herb.

Safety Information: Avoid completely if pregnant or nursing. Can be toxic if ingested.

FUN FACT:
Back in the days of yore, pennyroyal was also known as "pudding grass" for its use in a stuffing made of pennyroyal, honey, and pepper that was often used in hog's pudding.

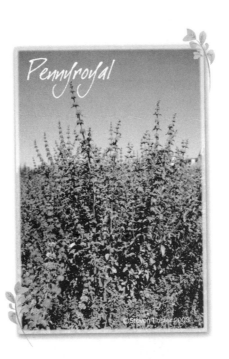

Pennyroyal

©Steven Foster 2003

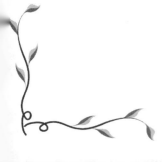

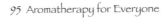

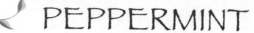

PEPPERMINT
(Mentha piperita)

Peppermint is one of the most useful and beloved essential oils. Refreshing, cooling, uplifting, and restoring, peppermint has a variety of therapeutic uses. Used extensively in both Eastern and Western medicine for everything from indigestion to diarrhea, headaches to tired feet, and toothaches to cramps. Peppermint is also a big favorite among the food industry, and can be found as a flavoring agent in gums, candy, ice cream, and pastries. However, peppermint really shines in aromatherapy, as its fresh, comforting scent soothes and relieves all sorts of ailments, both mental and physical.

Therapeutic uses: Apathy, arthritis, asthma, bad breath, back pain, bowel disorders, bronchitis, colds and flu, coughs, cramps, faintness, fatigue, flatulence, digestive problems, headaches, mental exhaustion, migraine, mouth or gum infections, muscular pain, nausea, poor circulation, sinus congestion, shock, sunburn, tired feet, travel sickness, vertigo.

Essential Oil Applications:

For apathy, fatigue, and mental exhaustion, use 2-3 drops in a diffuser.

For asthma, bronchitis, coughs, and sinus congestion, use 2-3 drops in a steam inhalation. Can also be used in a diffuser.

For bad breath and mouth or gum infections, use as a mouthwash.

To ease the discomfort of colds and flu accompanied by a headache, use 2-3 drops in a diffuser.

For cramps, tired feet, back pain, bowel disorders (inflammation, constipation, flatulence), headaches, mental exhaustion, muscular pain, rheumatism and arthritis, use 3-4 drops in 1 ounce of carrier oil and massage on body and/or affected areas.

For digestive problems and flatulence, use 2-3 drops in a carrier oil and massage on back. Can also be used in a compress.

For faintness, shock or vertigo, use 2-3 drops on a handkerchief and inhale periodically. Can also be used in a diffuser.

PEPPERMINT
(Mentha piperita)

To cool a fever, use 2-3 drops in a cold compress.

For headaches and migraine, use 2-3 drops in a diffuser.

To fight nausea, use 2-3 drops in a diffuser. Can also place a couple of drops on a handkerchief and inhale periodically.

To cool sunburn, add 2-3 drops to 2 tablespoons of liquid lanolin. Apply to affected area. Can also be used in a cold compress or in a carrier oil.

To alleviate travel sickness, use 2-3 drops on a handkerchief and inhale periodically.

Mixes well with: Basil, eucalyptus, geranium, grapefruit, juniper, lavender, lemon, myrrh, pine, rosemary, spearmint, tea tree, and wintergreen.

Extraction method: Steam distillation.

Parts used: Flowering herb.

Safety Information: Avoid if pregnant or breast feeding. Do not use on babies or small children. May cause irritation to sensitive skin, however it is rare. Do a patch test, first, before applying in large amounts. Do not use in baths. Should not be used in conjunction with homeopathic remedies, as it will act as an antidote.

FUN FACT:
It's believed that the genus Mentha was named for the mythological nymph Minthe, who, according to Roman legend, was seduced by Pluto, then turned into a plant by his jealous wife. Pluto then turned Minthe into an herb, to be valued by generations to come.

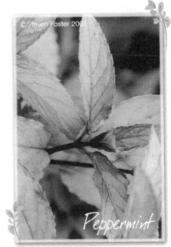

Peppermint

©Steven Foster 2008

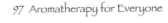

PINE NEEDLE
(Pinus sylvestris)

The fresh scent of pine awakens memories of crisp, winter days and of holidays past. Pine's uniquely comforting and invigorating scent has been used therapeutically for centuries. Ancient Greeks, Egyptians, and Arabians used pine in religious ceremonies, and also for conditions like bronchitis, tuberculosis, and pneumonia. Native Americans made a special brew with the needles, which was consumed to prevent scurvy. The Scandinavians used pine branches in saunas, and many cultures stuffed mattresses with pine needles to repel lice, fleas, and other insects. In fact, pine-needle mattresses are still used today in the Swiss Alps, however now their purpose is as a remedy for rheumatism. Pine oil is also a favorite in bath oils and foams (always with a carrier), because of both its fresh, lively scent and its antirheumatic properties.

Therapeutic uses: Asthma, athlete's foot, bronchitis, cellulite, colds and flu, coughs, cuts, cystitis, digestive problems, drowsiness, eczema, fatigue, gall bladder, hangover, nervous exhaustion, prostate problems, psoriasis, rheumatism, scabies, sciatica, sinus congestion, skin irritations, smoker's cough, sore throat, and sores.

Essential Oil Applications:

For asthma, bronchitis, coughs (including smoker's cough), or sore throat, use 2-3 drops in a steam inhalation. Can also use 2-3 drops in a diffuser or 8-10 drops in bath water.

For athlete's foot, cuts, eczema, psoriasis, scabies, sores, or other skin irritations, use 2-3 drops in 1 ounce of carrier oil and massage on area.

For cellulite, use 2-3 drops in a carrier oil and massage on affected area regularly. Can also use 8-10 drops in bath water.

For colds, flu, sinus congestion, and/or sore throats, use 2-3 drops in a diffuser or steam inhalation. Can also add 8-10 drops in bath water.

For cystitis or prostate problems, use 8-10 drops in bath water.

For digestive problems, use 2-3 drops in a steam inhalation. Can also mix 2-3 drops in 1 ounce of carrier oil, and rub on chest and lower back.

PINE NEEDLE
(Abies sirbirica)

To alleviate drowsiness or nervous exhaustion, use 2-3 drops in a diffuser.

For hangovers, use 2-3 drops in a hot or cold compress. Can also use 2-3 drops in a diffuser or 8-10 drops in bath water.

Mixes well with: Atlas cedarwood, cedarwood, citronella, clary sage, eucalyptus, frankincense, grapefruit, juniper, lavender, lemon, marjoram, myrrh, patchouli, peppermint, rosemary, sage, sandalwood, tea tree, and thyme.

Safety Information: Avoid if prone to allergic reactions. Avoid if diagnosed with high blood pressure. Should not be used on the skin of children or the elderly. Be sure to avoid oil from *Pinus pumilio* (dwarf pine).

Extraction method: Steam distillation.

Parts used: Needles, twigs, and buds.

FUN FACT:
Pine kernels were used in a bread eaten by ancient Romans, who believed it to be restorative.

(See Color Photo on Page 75)

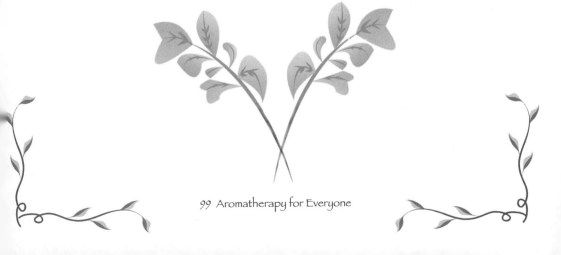

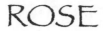

ROSE
(Rosa centifolia)

Fragrant, symbolic, and long-lasting, there is nothing in this world that can compare to the beauty and magnificence that is the rose. It has a long, layered history as rich as its fragrance. The Romans believed roses could prevent drunkenness, so they would scatter the petals at banquets. St. Dominic believed the Virgin Mary had visited him and gave him the first rosary, which was made with rose-scented beads. In the Middle Ages, roses were used as an ingredient in various healing balms used to treat ailments like lung disease and asthma. Symbolically, the rose represents transcendent desire in Sufi tradition, divine love in Christian tradition, and also represents the Rosacrucian order. Touted as a very feminine oil, rose oil is excellent for skin care and emotional balance. It's also very expensive: it takes 180 pounds of roses to make one ounce of rose oil. Therefore, it is not unusual to find it "cut" with another oil. The benefits are still in abundance, but the cost is more affordable!

Therapeutic uses: Allergies, anger, anxiety, asthma, circulation, constipation, coughs, depression, digestive system, grief, hay fever, headaches, irregular menstruation, jealousy, libido, migraine, nausea, nervous tension, postnatal depression, resentment, scar tissue, skin care, sore throats, stress, vomiting.

Essential Oil Applications:

For allergies and asthma, use 3-4 drops in a diffuser or 8-10 drops in bath water regularly.

To better bear anger, depression, grief, jealousy, and resentment, use 3-4 drops in a diffuser.

To alleviate anxiety and nervous tension, use 2-3 drops in a carrier oil and massage on body, or add 8-10 drops in bath water.

To stimulate circulation, use 3-4 drops in 1 ounce of carrier oil and massage on body. Can also add 8-10 drops in bath water.

For constipation, use 8-10 drops in bath water.

To fight off coughs and hay fever, use 8-10 drops in bath water. Can also mix 3-4 drops in 1 ounce of carrier oil and massage on body.

ROSE
(Rosa centifolia)

To ease headache and migraine, use 3-4 drops in a hot or cold compress (whichever works best for you). Can also use 3-4 drops in a diffuser.

To restore libido, use 6-8 drops in a bath. Can also use 2-3 drops in 1 ounce of carrier oil, and massage on body.

To ease nausea and vomiting, use 3-4 drops in a diffuser or 8-10 drops in bath water.

To alleviate postnatal depression, use 3-4 drops in a diffuser regularly. Can also mix 3-4 drops in 1 ounce of carrier oil for regular body massages.

For overall skin care and to help soften scar tissue, mix a few drops with a carrier oil and massage on body. Can also be mixed with water and applied to face; especially good for mature and/or sensitive skin.

Mixes well with: Bergamot, cinnamon, clary sage, clove, frankincense, geranium, ginger, jasmine, lemon, neroli, palmarosa, patchouli, sandalwood, tangerine, and ylang ylang.

Extraction method: Enfleurage and solvent extraction.

Parts used: Fresh flower heads.

Safety Information: Avoid during first four months of pregnancy.

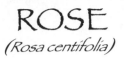

> ## FUN FACT:
> In Elizabethan times, rose-flavored food
> was all the rage.

(See Color Photo on Page 75)

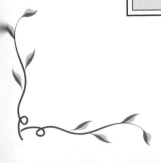

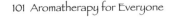

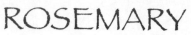

ROSEMARY
(Rosmarinus officinalis)

Rosemary was valued by the ancients of many cultures as a sacred plant that could impart peace to both the living and the dead. The Greeks burnt rosemary at shrines, and along with the Romans, considered it symbolic of remembrance and loyalty. During the Middle Ages, people wore rosemary garlands to bring them good luck and to protect them from evil spirits, magic, and witchcraft. It was also thought to help protect against the plague and other infectious illnesses. Nowadays rosemary is a popular culinary herb, and used in many delectable dishes. However, its charm isn't relegated to the kitchen: it's a powerful aromatic as well. Rosemary's fresh, minty, woody aroma can fight fatigue, uplift spirits, renew enthusiasm, and boost self-confidence. Rosemary also has antibacterial and antiseptic properties, making it a strong ally against colds, flu, and respiratory infections. Rosemary is a necessity for every aromatherapy kit.

Therapeutic uses: Acne, arthritis, asthma, back pain, cellulite, colds and flu, constipation, dandruff, depression, diarrhea, enthusiasm, fatigue, fluid retention, greasy hair and skin, headaches, memory enhancement, menstrual pain, migraines, muscular pain, nervous exhaustion, respiratory infections, rheumatism, self-confidence, sinus problems, stiff neck.

Essential Oil Applications:

For acne and greasy skin, use 2-3 drops on a wet cotton ball and dab on affected area.

For asthma and respiratory infections, use 2-3 drops in a steam inhalation. Can also use 2-3 drops in a diffuser or 8-10 drops in bath water.

For arthritis, back pain, muscular pain, rheumatism, or a stiff neck, use 2-3 drops in 1 ounce of carrier oil and massage on area.

For cellulite, use 2-3 drops in a carrier oil and massage on affected area regularly. Can also use 8-10 drops in bath water.

To help the body fight colds and flu, use 2-3 drops in a diffuser. Can also add 8-10 drops in bath water.

For constipation or diarrhea, use 8-10 drops in bath water. Can also mix 2-3 drops with 1 ounce of carrier oil and massage on lower back and abdomen area.

For dandruff and greasy hair, add 2-3 drops of oil to unscented conditioner.

ROSEMARY
(Rosmarinus officinalis)

Leave on 3-5 minutes, then rinse.

To relieve depression, fatigue, and nervous exhaustion, use 2-3 drops in a diffuser.

To restore enthusiasm and self-confidence, and enhance memory, use 2-3 drops in a diffuser.

To alleviate fluid retention and cellulite, use 8-10 drops in bath water regularly. Can also mix 2-3 drops to 1 ounce of carrier oil and massage on affected areas regularly.

For headaches and migraines, especially those related to gastric upset, use 2-3 drops in a hot or cold compress. Can also use 2-3 drops in a diffuser or 8-10 drops in bath water.

To alleviate menstrual pain, use 8-10 drops in bath water. Can also mix 2-3 drops in a carrier oil and massage on lower back and abdomen.

For sinus problems, use 2-3 drops in a steam inhalation.

Mixes well with: Atlas cedarwood, basil, bergamot, cedarwood, cinnamon, citronella, clove, eucalyptus, geranium, ginger, grapefruit, hyssop, juniper, lavender, lemon, lime, marjoram, myrrh, neroli, nutmeg, oregano, palmarosa, pennyroyal, peppermint, pine, rosewood, sage, spearmint, tangerine, tea tree, and thyme.

Extraction method: Steam distillation

Parts used: Fresh flowering tops or whole plant.

Safety Information: Avoid if pregnant. Do not use if diagnosed with epilepsy or high blood pressure. Do not rub or massage directly over or below varicose veins.

FUN FACT:
The British used to wear rosemary around their neck to prevent colds, and also wrapped it around their right arms to lift spirits.

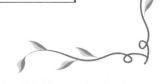

ROSEWOOD
(Aniba rosaeodora)

Rosewood is a beautiful, luxurious, amber-colored wood, often made into elegant furniture. The Japanese also use rosewood to make chopstix. Its warm, woody, spicy yet floral scent has made it a favorite component of many perfumes. Additionally, while rosewood may not be one of the most widely used essential oils, it has many highly valued aromatic properties. For centuries, the people of the Amazonian rainforest have used rosewood to heal wounds and also for various types of skin ailments. Rosewood can also boost the immune system, relieve headaches, and act as a deodorant. It also has tissue regeneration properties, making it a great combat tool against aging skin, wrinkles, and scars.

Therapeutic uses: acne, aging skin, colds, coughs, exhaustion, fever, infections, headaches, immune system, insect repellent, lethargy, libido, meditation, nausea, nervous tension, scars, stress-related problems, viruses, wounds, wrinkles.

Essential Oil Applications:

For acne, use 2-3 drops in a carrier oil and dab on affected area.

For aging skin, scars, and wrinkles, mix 2-3 drops with 2 tablespoons of liquid lanolin or a face and/or body cream, and apply to affected area.

To help the body deal with colds, infections, and viruses, and to boost the immune system, use 2-3 drops in a diffuser. Can also add 8-10 drops in bath water.

For ticklish coughs, use 2-3 drops in a steam inhalation. Can also add 8-10 drops in bath water.

To relieve exhaustion and lethargy, use 2-3 drops in a diffuser.

For fever, use 2-3 drops in a cold compress.

For headaches, especially those accompanied by nausea, use 2-3 drops in a hot or cold compress. Can also use 2-3 drops in a diffuser or 8-10 drops in bath water.

ROSEWOOD
(Aniba rosaeodora)

To repel insects, use 2-3 drops in a diffuser.

To restore libido, use 6-8 drops in a bath. Can also use 2-3 drops in 1 ounce of carrier oil, and massage on body.

For nervous tension, use 2-3 drops in a carrier oil and massage on body, or add 8-10 drops in bath water.

For wounds, use 2-3 drops in a cold compress after cleaning wound.

Mixes well with: Anise, Atlas cedarwood, geranium, grapefruit, jasmine, lemon, lime, marjoram, orange, patchouli, rosemary, sage, sandalwood, tangerine, tea tree, and ylang ylang.

Extraction method: Steam distillation.

Parts used: Wood chippings.

Safety Information: No special precautions required with rosewood.

FUN FACT:
Not only has rosewood been a favorite among French cabinet makers, but it was also used as handles for domestic utensils like brushes and knives.

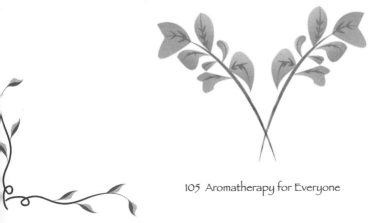

SAGE
(Salvia officinalis)
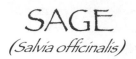

Throughout the ages, sage was considered to be a sacred herb, especially by the Romans, who believed a little bit of sage could cure just about everything. The Chinese also valued sage, and believed it to be a cure for sterility. This savory herb found its way into the kitchen, and was used to flavor meats and other dishes. As an aromatic, sage has a variety of therapeutic uses, from promoting respiratory health to strengthening memory. Sage is also a popular fragrance in perfumes and colognes, especially men's products. It can also be found in soaps, shampoos, detergents, and antiperspirants, as well as mouthwashes, gargles and toothpastes. To cap it all off, sage is also a source of natural antioxidants *(although ingesting it in essential oil form is not recommended)*. There are many different varieties of sage, however salvia officinalis is used in aromatherapy because it is both commercially and therapeutically important. It's still current in the British Herbal Pharmacopoeia, and especially wonderful when blended with citrus essential oils.

Therapeutic uses: Appetite, arthritis, bronchitis, constipation, coughs, fluid retention, indigestion, low blood pressure, memory, menopause, menstruation, over-exercised muscles, respiratory problems, rheumatism, trauma.

Essential Oil Applications:

To restore appetite, use 2-3 drops in a diffuser.

For arthritis, over-exercised muscles, and rheumatism, use 2-3 drops in one ounce of carrier oil and massage on affected areas.

For bronchitis, coughs, and other respiratory problems, use 2-3 drops in a steam inhalation. Can also use 2-3 drops in a diffuser.

For constipation, use 8-10 drops in bath water.

To alleviate fluid retention, use 2-3 drops in one ounce of carrier oil, and massage on affected areas, such as legs. Can also use 8-10 drops in bath water.

For indigestion, use 2-3 drops in steam inhalation, or 8-10 drops in bath water.

SAGE
(Salvia officinalis)

For flatulence, use 2-3 drops in a steam inhalation or diffuser.

To help fight low blood pressure, use 2-3 drops in diffuser or steam inhalation regularly.

To strengthen memory, use 2-3 drops in a diffuser regularly.

To alleviate menopausal discomfort such as hot flashes and night sweats, and to balance nerves, use 2-3 drops in a diffuser nightly.

To help with scanty periods and painful menstruation, use 8-10 drops in bath water.

To restore a sense of balance and calmness after trauma, especially trauma that continues to haunt you after a long period of time, use 2-3 drops in a diffuser nightly until a sense of balance is restored.

Mixes well with: Bergamot, grapefruit, hyssop, lavender, lemon, lime, orange, pennyroyal, pine, rosemary, rosewood, and tangerine.

Extraction method: Steam distillation

Parts used: Dried leaves

Safety Information: Avoid during pregnancy, and also if breastfeeding. If diagnosed with epilepsy or high blood pressure small amounts are fine, however it is safest to avoid it. Sage should also not be used on babies or small children.

FUN FACT:
During the Middle Ages, the actual herb – and not the oil – was used to clean gums.

©Steven Foster 2003

Sage

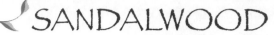

SANDALWOOD
(Santalum album)

Sandalwood is one of the oldest substances used in perfumes and other toiletries (over 4,000 years). It has a sensual, musky scent, reminiscent of the Orient. Besides its presence in many perfumes, sandalwood is also a big part of numerous different types of religious and cultural ceremonies and traditions. Many Muslims burn sandalwood at the feet of the recently deceased to hasten their soul to heaven. In Japan, sandalwood is burned in Shinto ceremonies and at Buddhist shrines, and ancient Egyptians used it in the embalming process. Unfortunately its popularity has contributed to the fact that sandalwood trees are now almost extinct, and are farmed on plantations exclusively for the production of their essential oil.

Therapeutic uses: Acne, anxiety, aphrodisiac, bladder infections, boils, chapped, dry, or cracked skin, chest infections, cystitis, diarrhea, dandruff, depression, dry coughs, dry eczema, heartburn, insect repellent, insomnia, nervous tension, razor rash, sore throat.

Essential Oil Applications:

For acne, boils, and eczema, mix 2-3 drops with a carrier oil and dab on affected area. Can also be used neat. (Essential oils are highly concentrated plant oils. Read and follow instructions for use carefully.)

For anxiety, depression, insomnia, and nervous tension, use 2-3 drops in an diffuser. Can also add 8-10 drops to bath water.

As an aphrodisiac, use 2-3 drops in a diffuser. Can also add 8-10 drops to bath water.

For bladder infections or cystitis, use 8-10 drops in bath water. Can also add 2-3 drops to a carrier oil and massage on lower back and abdomen area.

For chapped, dry, or cracked skin, mix 2-3 drops with 2 tablespoons of liquid lanolin. Rub into affected areas.

For dandruff, mix a 2-3 drops in unscented conditioner and apply to scalp. Leave on for 3-5 minutes, then rinse.

SANDALWOOD
(Santalum album)

For diarrhea, add 8-10 drops in bath water and take a nice, long soak. Can also add 2-3 drops to a carrier oil and massage into lower back and abdomen area.

For chest infections or dry cough, use 2-3 drops in a steam inhalation. Can also use 2-3 drops in a diffuser or 8-10 drops in bath water.

For heartburn, use 2-3 drops in 1 ounce of carrier oil and rub on chest. Can also use 8-10 drops in bath water or 2-3 drops in a diffuser.

As an insect repellent, use 2-3 drops in a diffuser.

For razor rash, put 2-3 drops on a wet cotton ball and dab on skin.

For a sore throat, apply neat to throat area. (Essential oils are highly concentrated plant oils. Read and follow instructions for use carefully.)

Mixes well with: Anise, basil, bergamot, cedarwood, clove, frankincense, geranium, ginger, grapefruit, jasmine, juniper, lavender, lemon, lime, myrrh, neroli, orange, palmarosa, patchouli, pine, rose, rosewood, tangerine, and ylang ylang.

Extraction method: Water or steam distillation.

Parts used: Heartwood and roots.

Safety Information: The scent of sandalwood can linger on clothing, even after washing.

FUN FACT:
Sandalwood is used in a Hindu purification ceremony that takes place on the last day of the year to wash away sins.

(See Color Photo on Page 76)

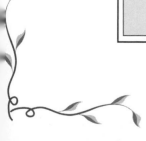

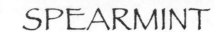

SPEARMINT
(Mentha spicata)

Spearmint is a favorite flavor for gums and mints because of its refreshing and cleansing taste. However, this herb has been used for centuries for its therapeutic properties. The Greeks not only used it to scent their bath water, but as a restorative as well. In medieval times, spearmint was used to heal sore gums and whiten teeth. Today, spearmint is a favorite flavoring agent, and it is also a valued aromatic. Spearmint helps with digestive problems, headaches, respiratory health , and skin problems. Its fresh, minty aroma is invigorating and energizing, making it a wonderful scent to come home to and recharge after a demanding, stressful day.

Therapeutic uses: Acne, asthma, bronchitis, colds and flu, congested skin, dermatitis, fatigue, fever, flatulence, headache, migraine, nausea, nervous strain, sinusitis, sore gums, stress, vomiting.

Essential Oil Applications:

For acne or congested skin, use 2-3 drops in a carrier oil and dab on affected area.

For asthma, bronchitis, and sinusitis, use 2-3 drops in a steam inhalation. Can also use 2-3 drops in a diffuser.

For colds, fever, and flu, use 2-3 drops cold compress for fever, or hot compress for colds and flu. Can also add 8-10 drops in bath water. Spearmint is also good in a sickroom to help reenergize; 2-3 drops in a diffuser will help accomplish that.

To relieve fatigue, nervous strain, and stress, use 2-3 drops in a diffuser.

For flatulence, use 2-3 drops in a steam inhalation or diffuser.

For headaches and migraines, use 2-3 drops in a diffuser or steam inhalation. Can also use 2-3 drops in an ounce of carrier oil and massage on temples, or 8-10 drops in bath water.

To help alleviate the pain of sore gums, use in a homemade mouthwash.

SPEARMINT
(Mentha spicata)

For vomiting, use 2-3 drops in a steam inhalation to help calm the system.

Mixes well with: Basil, eucalyptus, ginger, lavender, myrrh, peppermint, rosemary, and wintergreen.

Extraction method: Steam distillation.

Parts used: Fresh flowering tops or whole plant.

Safety Information: Not compatible with homeopathic treatment.

> ## FUN FACT:
> In ancient times, spearmint was renowned for curing sexually transmitted diseases, however, modern medical technology has not proven that spearmint has this power. In other words, kids, don't try this treatment at home!

(See Color Photo on Page 76)

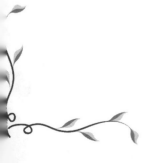

TANGERINE
(Citrus reticulata)

Tangerines are much more than a delicious, exotic treat. These fabulous fruits have been used throughout the ages for skin care, digestive health, and system balancing. Their warm, sweet, fresh, and lively scent is especially captivating to children and pregnant women. The French regard tangerine oil as a safe remedy for children suffering from indigestion and hiccoughs. Tangerine oil is also known to inspire, strengthen, and uplift spirits. This essential oil helps combat PMS, promotes healthy digestion, and can help reduce scars and stretch marks. It also supports the lymphatic, circulatory, and immune systems. While some may find it similar to orange oil, tangerine oil has its own unique, comforting, and sparkling aroma, and should not be replaced by its citrus sister.

Therapeutic uses: Acne, anxiety, cellulite, congested skin, cramped muscles, constipation, diarrhea, digestion, fear, flatulence, hiccoughs, hyperactivity, insomnia, intestinal problems, irritability, muscle cramps, oily skin, premenstrual syndrome, restlessness, sadness, scars, stretch marks, tension, water retention.

Essential Oil Applications:

For acne, congested or oily skin, scars, and stretch marks, use 2-3 drops in a carrier oil and massage on affected areas. Can also use 8-10 drops in bath water.

To alleviate anxiety, fear, hyperactivity, insomnia, irritability, PMS symptoms, restlessness, sadness, and tension, use 2-3 drops in a diffuser. Can also add 8-10 drops in bath water.

For cellulite and water retention, use 2-3 drops in one ounce of carrier oil and massage on affected area regularly. Can also use 8-10 drops in bath water.

To relieve constipation, flatulence, and/or diarrhea, use 8-10 drops in bath water. Can also use 2-3 drops in a diffuser.

To relieve hiccoughs, use 2-3 drops in a steam inhalation.

To relieve muscle cramps, use 2-3 drops in one ounce of carrier oil and massage on affected area. Can also use in a hot compress.

TANGERINE
(Citrus reticulata)

To maintain a healthy digestive system, mix 2-3 drops in a carrier oil and gently massage on stomach in a clockwise motion. Do this regularly.

Mixes well with: Anise, basil, bergamot, cinnamon, clary sage, clove, frankincense, geranium, ginger, grapefruit, hyssop, juniper, lavender, lemon, lime, marjoram, myrrh, neroli, nutmeg, palmarosa, patchouli, rose, rosemary, rosewood, sage, sandalwood, tea tree, and ylang ylang.

Extraction method: Cold expression.

Parts used: Outer peel.

Safety Information: May be phototoxic; do not use on skin exposed to direct sunlight.

FUN FACT:
In the days of simpler gift giving, tangerines were a favorite stocking stuffer, and delighted both the giver and the receiver.

(See Color Photo on Page 76)

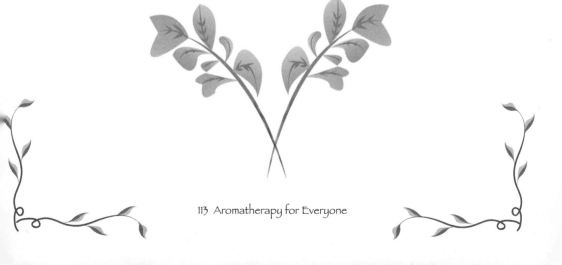

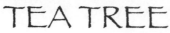

TEA TREE
(Melaleuca alternifolia)

Well-known for its antiseptic and germicidal properties, tea tree oil has been used therapeutically by the aboriginal people of Australia for centuries. Named by Captain Cook's crew, it was introduced to Europe around 1927. During World War II, Australian soldiers carried tea tree oil in their first-aid kits as a treatment for skin injuries. Even though tea tree oil has a long history of use therapeutically, it is a relatively new addition to aromatherapy. Despite being the new kid on the block, tea tree oil has become a staple for many aromatherapists around the world because of its versatility and wide-reaching benefits.

Therapeutic uses: Acne, asthma, athlete's foot, blemishes from chicken pox and shingles, blisters, bronchitis, burns, chilblains, cold sores, colds and flu, coughs, cracked and rough skin, dandruff, debilitating illnesses, fever, flu, insect bites, operation recovery, repeated infections, sinusitis, sunburn, varicose veins, warts, whooping cough.

Essential Oil Applications:

For acne, athlete's foot, blemishes from chicken pox and shingles, blisters, burns, chilblains, cold sores, cracked and rough skin, dandruff, insect bites, sunburn, varicose veins, and warts, can apply neat to affected area (avoid surrounding area). Can also be used with water in a compress, or in a hair rinse. Be sure to carry out a patch test first before applying neat on skin.

For asthma, bronchitis, coughs, sinusitis, and whooping cough, use 8-10 drops in bath water. Can also use 2-3 drops in one ounce of carrier oil and massage gently on chest and back.

For colds and flu, use 2-3 drops in a diffuser. Can also use 8-10 drops in in bath water.

For fever, use 3-5 drops in a cold compress.

To help the body throw off repeated infections and debilitating illnesses, use 2-3 drops in a diffuser regularly. Can also use 2-3 drops in one ounce of carrier oil and massage regularly on body.

TEA TREE
(Melaleuca alternifolia)

To help prepare the body before an operation, mix 2-3 drops in carrier oil and massage on body. To help relieve postoperative shock, use in the same way, carefully avoiding the operation wound or scar.

Mixes well with: Basil, bergamot, citronella, clary sage, clove, eucalyptus, geranium, ginger, juniper, lavender, lemon, marjoram, myrrh, nutmeg, oregano, peppermint, pine, rosemary, rosewood, tangerine, tea tree, thyme, and ylang ylang.

Extraction method: Steam or water distillation.

Parts used: Leaves and twigs.

Safety Information: Can be used neat, however it's best to do a patch test first. Limit usage to the problem area, and avoid the surrounding skin. Do not massage directly on or below a varicose vein.

FUN FACT:
During World War II, Australian cutters and producers of tea tree oil were exempt from military service until enough of this precious essential oil was accumulated for use in first-aid kits.

(See Color Photo on Page 76)

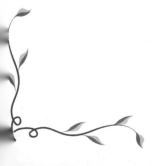

THYME
(Thymus vulgaris)

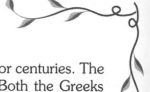

Warm and spicy, thyme has been a beloved aromatic for centuries. The ancient Greeks burned it as incense inside temples. Both the Greeks and the Romans used thyme to flavor cheese and liquor. The Egyptians used it in the embalming process. Thyme was also a symbol of courage, and in the Middle Ages, knights wore scarves embroidered with a sprig of thyme. A soup of beer and thyme was consumed to help overcome shyness. The Scots used to make a tea of wild thyme, and believed that drinking it would boost courage and strength, plus prevent nightmares. Now, thyme is most popular in the kitchen, however, aromatherapists everywhere know of its therapeutic value and employ it in their practices.

Therapeutic uses: Acne, arthritis, asthma, bronchitis, bruises, burns, chills, colds and flu, coughs, cuts, dermatitis, eczema, infectious diseases, insect bites, gout, gum infections, headaches, insomnia, laryngitis, mucuous congestion, muscular aches and pains, physical exhaustion, poor circulation, oily skin, rheumatism, sinusitis, sore throat, sports injuries, sprains, stress-related complaints, tonsillitis, warts.

Essential Oil Applications:

For acne, bruises, burns, cuts, eczema, insect bites, oily skin, and warts, place 2-3 drops on a cotton ball and dab on affected area.

For arthritis, gout, muscle aches and pains, sports injuries, sprains, and rheumatism, use 2-3 drops in a carrier oil and massage on affected area.

For asthma, bronchitis, and coughs, use 2-3 drops in 1 ounce of carrier oil and rub on chest and throat. Can also use 2-3 drops in a steam inhalation.

For chills associated with colds or flu, use 2-3 drops in 1 ounce of carrier oil and massage on body.

For colds, flu, mucous infections, and sinusitis, use 2-3 drops in a steam inhalation.

For gum infections, sore throat, and tonsillitis, use diluted in a gargle or mouthwash.

THYME
(Thymus vulgaris)

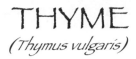

For insomnia, physical exhaustion, and stress-related complaints, use 2-3 drops in a diffuser.

For headaches, use 2-3 drops in 1 ounce of carrier oil and massage on temples and neck. Can also be used in a hot or cold compress.

To combat poor circulation, use 2-3 drops in 1 ounce of carrier oil and massage on body.

Mixes well with: Bergamot, cinnamon, clary sage, eucalyptus, geranium, grapefruit, lavender, lemon, marjoram, myrrh, oregano, palmarosa, pine, rosemary, tea tree, and wintergreen.

Extraction method: Steam or water distillation.

Parts used: Flowering tops and fresh or partially dried leaves..

Safety Information: Avoid if diagnosed with high blood pressure. Not to be used in baths. Some highly sensitive people could have a reaction, so do a patch test, first, before using neat on skin. (Essential oils are highly concentrated plant oils. Read and follow instructions for use carefully.)

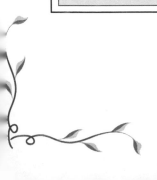

FUN FACT:
Fairies were once thought to
live in beds of thyme.
(And who knows for sure?
Maybe they do!)

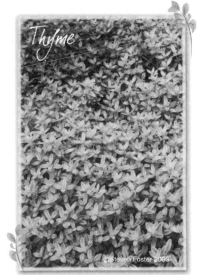

Thyme

WINTERGREEN
(Gaultheria procumbens)

Traditionally, wintergreen has been used for centuries for muscle aches and pains, arthritis, and rheumatism. While its aroma is on the minty side, it has a warming quality that makes it perfect for relieving the aches and pains associated with those problems. Native Americans used crushed leaves to alleviate the pain of strained muscles, and also as an anti-inflammatory. What many may not realize is wintergreen is often used in perfumery applications, especially fragrances that possess a forest-type scent. And while wintergreen is a well-known flavoring agent for toothpastes, chewing gum, and candy, it is also used in many soft drinks, like root beer. And in what may be the biggest surprise to consumers everywhere, wintergreen is used in the world's most recognized soft drink: Coca-Cola. Its use in aromatherapy is sweet as well, as it provides sweet relief to many who suffer from the aches and pains of ailments like arthritis.

Therapeutic uses: Acne, arthritis, back pain, cellulitis, fever, fibromylagia, headaches, lumbago, muscle aches and pains, oily skin, rheumatism, sciatica, sore throats.

Essential Oil Applications:

For arthritis, cellulitis, fibromylagia, lumbago, muscle aches and pains, rheumatism, and sciatica, use 2-3 drops in one ounce of carrier oil and massage on affected areas.

For acne and oily skin, mix 2-3 drops in one ounce of carrier oil and dab on affected area with a cotton ball or swab.

For headaches or fever, use 2-3 drops in a cold compress.

For sore throats, mix 2-3 drops in one ounce of carrier oil and massage on throat.

Mixes well with: Oregano, peppermint, spearmint, thyme, and ylang ylang.

Extraction method: Steam or water distillation.

WINTERGREEN
(Gaultheria procumbens)

Parts used: Leaves.

Safety Information: Avoid if pregnant. Only for topical use, and only if diluted. Not for use on children under 12.

FUN FACT:
During the Revolutionary War, wintergreen leaves were used as tea because black tea was so highly taxed.

(See Color Photo on Page 76)

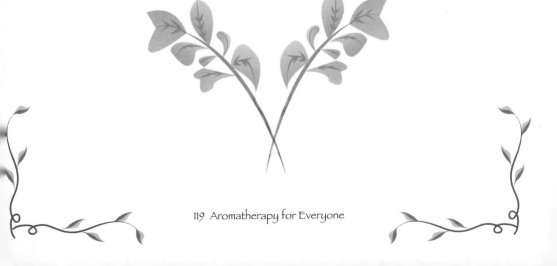

YLANG-YLANG
(Canaga odorata)

Exotic. Mysterious. Spicy. Those three words describe ylang ylang to a "T." Ylang ylang's aroma can both uplift and relax. It's been around for centuries, and has been most frequently used as an aphrodisiac, yet it has many other stimulating qualities as well. Victorians used it to stimulate the scalp to encourage hair growth. The Chinese used it for circulatory health and to balance the heart. Early 20th century researchers discovered ylang ylang oil was effective against malaria, typhus, and various intestinal infections. Around the same time, researchers also recognized ylang ylang had a calming effect on the heart. Today, ylang ylang is a treasured essential oil, and is actually more powerful when combined with other oils.

Therapeutic uses: Anxiety, aphrodisiac, depression, dry skin, fear, frigidity, high blood pressure, impotence, insomnia, intestinal infections and upsets, oily skin, panic, physical exhaustion, postnatal depression, rapid breathing, rapid heartbeat, shock, stomach upsets and mild food poisoning, stress, tension.

Essential Oil Applications:

To relieve anxiety, circulatory health, depression, hair growth, insomnia, panic, physical exhaustion, postnatal depression, rapid breathing and/or heartbeat, shock, stress, and tension, use 2-3 drops in a diffuser. Can also add 8-10 drops in bath water.

As an aphrodisiac, use 2-3 drops in a diffuser or 8-10 drops in bath water.

To help alleviate frigidity or impotence, use 2-3 drops in a diffuser or 8-10 drops in bath water.

For circulatory health, mix 2-3 drops in 1 ounce of carrier oil and massage on body.

To stimulate hair growth, mix with a carrier oil and massage into scalp. Leave on 20 minutes, shampoo out.

To lower high blood pressure, use 2-3 drops in a diffuser or steam inhalation regularly.

YLANG-YLANG
(Canaga odorata)

To regulate sebum production (good for either oily or dry skin) use 2-3 drops on a damp cotton ball and apply to affected area.

For stomach upsets or mild food poisoning, mix 2-3 drops in a carrier oil and massage gently on stomach area.

Mixes well with: Allspice, Atlas cedarwood, bergamot, cinnamon, frankincense, geranium, ginger, grapefruit, jasmine, lavender, lemon, lime, marjoram, myrrh, neroli, orange, palmarosa, patchouli, rose, rosewood, sandalwood, tangerine, tea tree, and wintergreen.

Extraction method: Water or steam distillation.

Parts used: Fresh, fully-developed flowers.

Safety Information: Use in small qualities, used too frequently or in high doses could cause headaches or nausea in some people. Do not use on inflamed skin, or skin affected by dermatitis.

FUN FACT:
Indonesians spread ylang-ylang petals on
the bed of newly wedded couples.

(See Color Photo on Page 76)

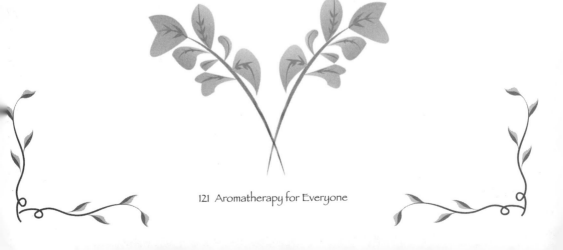

BIOGRAPHIES

Pamela Pierson

Pamela Pierson is a freelancer who has been writing about health and nutrition issues for a decade. Although she started out her adult life as a soldier in the United States Army, she discovered a flair and a love for writing as she constantly filed missives homeward. After thirteen years in the service, she pursued writing and discovered a love for creative non-fiction, with a particular fancy for health and nutrition issues. A California native, she now lives in Sparks, Nevada with her long-time partner, Todd, two purrfectly good cats, and Glindy the dog.

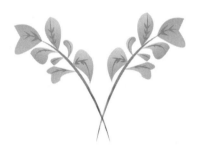

Mary Shipley

Mary Shipley has been involved with natural care and herbal healing since the early 70's. Following the loss of her 3-year-old son to meningitis, she vowed to become more knowledgeable of the body and its systems. Although Mary studied Nursing at the College of DuPage (Illinois), earned an Associate's of Science Degree, and a BA from Northern Illinois University, she's come to believe that modern medicine falls short. She knew that in the field of Natural Health there were cures and ways to maintain one's health that are completely ignored in most traditional textbooks. For the past 7 years Mary has worked with NOW Foods. She is also currently working on her Masters Degree in Natural Health, through Clayton College. Upon graduation she intends to continue on to obtain her PhD. In her spare time Mary's an active organic gardener, growing many of her own herbs to support a fragrant and healthy lifestyle.

BIBLIOGRAPHY

Balch, Phyllis C.N.C. *Prescription For Herbal Healing*. Avery, A Member Of Penguin Putnam Inc. New York. 2002.

Berwick, Ann. *Aromatherapy A Holistic Guide: Balance the Body and Soul with Essential Oils*, Publisher: St. Paul, Minn USA: Llewellyn, c1994

Byers, Dorie. *Natural Body Basics*. Gooseberry Hill Publications, Inc., Bargersville, Indiana 1996.

Byers, Dorie R.N. *Natural Beauty Basics*. Vital Health Publishing, Bloomingdale, IL 2001.

Cooksley, Valerie Gennari R.N. *Healing Home Spa*. Prentice Hall Press, New York. 2003.

Dana, Mrs. William Star. *How To Know The Wild Flowers*. Houghton Mifflin Company, Boston. 1989.

Drs. Ali, Grant, Nakla. Patel And Vegotsky. *The Tea Tree Oil Bible*. Ages Publications, Niagara Falls, New York & Toronto, Ontario. 1999.

Edwards, Victoria H. *The Aromatherapy Companion*. Storey Books, North Adams, Ma. 1999.

Fischer-Rizzi, Susanne. *Complete Aromatherapy Handbook: Essential Oils for Radiant Health*, Publisher: New York, Sterling Pub. Co., c1990

Gattefoss`e, Ren`e-maurice. *Gattefoss`e's Aromatheraphy*. The C.W. Daniel Company Limited. 1937.

Kaminski, Patricia. *Flowers That Heal, How To Use Flower Essences*. Newleaf. Goldenbridge, Dublin. 1998.

Lavabre, Marcel. *Aromatherapy Workbook*. Healing Arts Press, Rochester, Vermont. 1990.

BIBLIOGRAPHY

Lawless, Julia. *Rose Oil*. Thorsons Publishers, Great Britain. 1995.

Lawless, Julia. *The Illustrated Encyclopedia to Essential Oils: The Complete Guide to the Use of Oils in Aromatherapy*, Publisher: Shaftsberry, Eng; Rockport, Mass.: Element, c1995

Maindells, Earl R. PH., Ph.d. *Herb Bible*. A Fireside Book Published By Simon & Schuster. New York, London, Toronto, Sydney, Toko, Singapore. 1992.

Metcalfe, Joannah. *Culpepper Guides Herbs And Aromatherapy*. Bloomsberry Book, London. 1989.

Nuzzi, Debra. *Herbal Reference Guide*. The Crossing Press, Freedom Ca. 1992.

Richard, David. *Anoint Yourself With Oil*. Vital Health Publishing, Bloomingdale, IL. 1997.

Schiller, David & Carol. *Aromatherapy Oils: A Complete Guide*, Publisher: New York: Sterling Pub. Co., c1996

Tisserand, Robert B. *The Art Of Aromatherapy*. Healing Arts Press. 1977.

Walters, Clare. *Aromatherapy: An Illustrated Guide*, Publisher: Boston: Element c1998

Whichello Brown, Denise. *Aromatherapy* Publisher: Lincolnwood ILL : NTC Publishing c1996

Wilson, Roberta. *Aromatherapy: Essential Oils For Vibrant Health And Beauty*. Avery. New York. 2002.

Worwood, Valerie Ann. *The Complete Book of Essential Oils and Aromatherapy* Publisher: San Rafael Calif.: New World Library, c1991

INDEX

RESOURCES

How To Locate and Purchase Essential Oils

There are various companies in the marketplace that sell essential oils. Some are more reputable than others. The following are oils that we are familiar with and trust, arranged by ease of availability.

NOW Foods has both 100% Pure and 100% Organic lines. They can be found at health food stores across the country, or special ordered through any store that carries NOW nutritional supplements. Go to their website to find a store near you.

Frontier/Aura Cacia has both 100% Pure and 100% Organic lines. They can be found at health food stores across the country, or ordered online.

Aroma Land oils are carried by select retailers and are sold through catalogs and online.

Aroma Vera oils are carried by select retailers and are sold through catalogs and online. This is a good source for some of the more exotic oils.

Young Living makes and distributes high quality therapeutic grade oils, but are sold mainly through multi-level marketing which makes them somewhat less available to the general consumer.

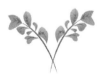

NOW Foods
www.nowfoods.com
1.888.669.3663

Aroma Vera
www.aromavera.com
1.800.669.9514

AromaLand
www.aromaland.com
1.800.933.5267

Frontier or Aura Cacia
www.frontiercoop.com
1.800.669.3275

Young Living
www.youngliving.com
1.800.371.2928

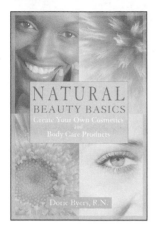

NATURAL BEAUTY BASICS
Create Your Own Cosmetics and Body Care Products
Dorie Byers, RN

Every day, television and magazine ads tell us that beautiful skin and hair are available only through the use of costly brand-name products. But the fact is that you can attain a radiant appearance by using products made inexpensively at home. That's what *Natural Beauty Basics* is all about. The author guides you to the equipment and ingredients you'll need to make your own products, and then presents easy-to-follow recipes for over 150 all-natural, effective, allergen-free creams, shampoos, soaps, and more.

$14.95 • 208 pages • 6 x 9-inch paperback • ISBN 978-1-890612-19-1

WHAT YOU MUST KNOW ABOUT VITAMINS, MINERALS, HERBS & MORE
Choosing the Nutrients That Are Right for You
Pamela Wartian Smith, MD, MPH

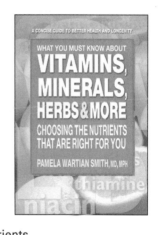

Almost 75 percent of your health and life expectancy is based on lifestyle, environment, and nutrition. Yet even if you follow a sound diet, you are probably not getting all the nutrients you need to prevent disease. In *What You Must Know About Vitamins, Minerals, Herbs & More,* Dr. Pamela Smith explains how you can restore and maintain health through the wise use of nutrients.

Part One of this easy-to-use guide discusses the individual nutrients necessary for good health. Part Two offers personalized nutritional programs for people with a wide variety of health concerns. People without prior medical problems can look to Part Three for their supplementation plans. Whether you want to maintain good health or you are trying to overcome a medical condition, *What You Must Know About Vitamins, Minerals, Herbs & More* can help you make the best choices for the well-being of you and your family.

$15.95 • 448 pages • 6 x 9-inch paperback • ISBN 978-0-7570-0233-5

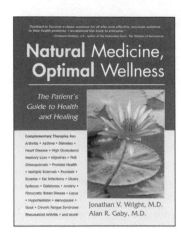

NATURAL MEDICINE, OPTIMAL WELLNESS
The Patient's Guide to Health and Healing
Jonathan V. Wright, MD, and Alan R. Gaby, MD

Imagine having holistic physicians at your fingertips to answer your medical questions. With *Natural Medicine, Optimal Wellness,* you do. For each condition, you'll sit in on a consultation between Dr. Jonathan Wright and a patient seeking advice. By the conclusion of each visit, you'll have a complete understanding of why Dr. Wright prescribes particular natural treatments. Then, in a separate commentary, Dr. Alan Gaby follows up with an analysis of the scientific evidence behind the treatments discussed, enabling you to make informed decisions about your health.

If you wish to receive the best of care from the best of physicians, *Natural Medicine, Optimal Wellness* is the natural choice for your personal library of health and wellness books.

$21.95 • 400 pages • 8.5 x 11-inch paperback • ISBN 978-1-890612-50-4

HEALING MUSHROOMS
Effective Treatments for Today's Illnesses
Georges M. Halpern, MD, PhD

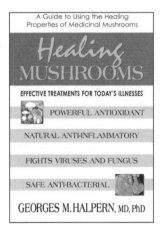

This easy-to-use guide begins by describing how ancient cultures utilized mushrooms to combat disease. It then explains how modern science has refocused its attention on the healing properties of mushrooms and, along the way, discovered wonderful new properties. Included are chapters that examine the folklore, health benefits, and culinary uses of mushrooms, including detailed instructions for buying, storing, and using eight major varieties of this valuable food.

From their use as a cholesterol-lowering agent to their promise of reversing Alzheimer's, mushrooms are among nature's greatest wonders. Let *Healing Mushrooms* change the way you think about this marvelous medicinal.

$15.95 • 192 pages • 6 x 9-inch paperback • ISBN 978-0-7570-0196-3

The Acid-Alkaline Food Guide
A Quick Reference to Foods & Their Effect on pH Levels
Dr. Susan E. Brown and Larry Trivieri, Jr.

In the last few years, researchers around the world have reported the importance of acid-alkaline balance to good health. While thousands of people are trying to balance their body's pH level, until now, they have had to rely on guides containing only a small number of foods. *The Acid-Alkaline Food Guide* is a complete resource for people who want to widen their food choices.

The book begins by explaining how the acid-alkaline environment of the body is influenced by foods. It then presents a list of thousands of foods—single foods, combination foods, and even fast foods—and their acid-alkaline effects. *The Acid-Alkaline Food Guide* will quickly become the resource you turn to at home, in restaurants, and whenever you want to select a food that can help you reach your health and dietary goals.

$7.95 • 208 pages • 4 x 7-inch mass paperback • ISBN 978-0-7570-0280-9

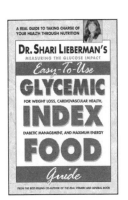

Glycemic Index Food Guide
For Weight Loss, Cardiovascular Health, Diabetic Management, and Maximum Energy
Dr. Shari Lieberman

The glycemic index (GI) is an important nutritional tool. By indicating how quickly a given food triggers a rise in blood sugar, the GI enables you to choose foods that can help you manage a variety of conditions and improve your overall health.

Written by leading nutritionist Dr. Shari Lieberman, this book was designed as an easy-to-use guide to the glycemic index. The book first answers commonly asked questions, ensuring that you truly understand the GI and know how to use it. It then provides both the glycemic index and the glycemic load of hundreds of foods and beverages, including raw foods, cooked foods, and many combination and prepared foods. Whether you are interested in controlling your glucose levels to manage your diabetes, lose weight, increase your heart health, or simply enhance your well-being, the *Glycemic Index Food Guide* is the best place to start.

$7.95 • 160 pages • 4 x 7-inch mass paperback • ISBN 978-0-7570-0245-8

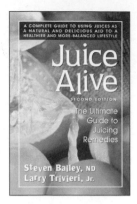

JUICE ALIVE, SECOND EDITION
The Ultimate Guide to Juicing Remedies
Steven Bailey, ND, and Larry Trivieri, Jr.

The world of fresh juices offers a powerhouse of antioxidants, vitamins, minerals, and enzymes. The trick is knowing which juices can best serve your needs. In this easy-to-use guide, health experts Dr. Steven Bailey and Larry Trivieri, Jr. tell you everything you need to know to maximize the benefits and tastes of juice.

The book begins with a look at the history of juicing. It then examines the many components that make fresh juice truly good for you—good for weight loss and so much more. Next, it offers practical advice about the types of juices available, as well as buying and storing tips for produce. The second half of the book begins with an important chart that matches up common ailments with the most appropriate juices, followed by over 100 delicious juice recipes. Let *Juice Alive* introduce you to a world bursting with the incomparable tastes and benefits of fresh juice.

$14.95 • 272 pages • 6 x 9-inch paperback • ISBN 978-0-7570-0266-3

SUICIDE BY SUGAR
A Startling Look at Our #1 National Addiction
Nancy Appleton, PhD, and G.N. Jacobs

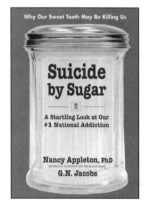

It is a dangerous, addictive white powder that can be found in abundance throughout this country. It is not illegal. In fact, it is available near playgrounds, schools, and vacation spots, and once we are hooked on it, the cravings can be overwhelming. This white substance of abuse is sugar.

Over two decades ago, Nancy Appleton's *Lick the Sugar Habit* exposed the dangers of America's high-sugar diet. Now, *Suicide by Sugar* presents a broader view of the problems caused by our favorite ingredient. The authors offer startling facts linking a range of disorders—from dementia to obesity—to our growing sugar addiction. Rounding out the book is a sound diet plan along with a number of recipes for sweet, delectable dishes.

Suicide by Sugar shines a bright light on our nation's addiction and helps us begin the journey toward health.

$15.95 • 192 pages • 6 x 9-inch paperback • ISBN 978-0-7570-0306-6

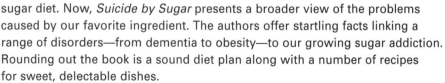

**For more information about our books,
visit our website at www.squareonepublishers.com**